Best Books For Young Adults, 1979.

W9-BBE-605

Scott Was Here

Scott
Was Here
ELAINE IPSWITCH

DELACORTE PRESS/NEW YORK

Published by
Delacorte Press
1 Dag Hammarskjold Plaza
New York, N.Y. 10017

Manufactured in the United States of America
First printing

Library of Congress Cataloging in Publication Data

Ipswitch, Elaine.
    Scott was here.

    1. Hodgkin's disease—Biography. 2. Ipswitch,
Scott, 1961–1976. I. Title.
RC644.I67   362.1'9'642   [B]   78–13969

ISBN 0-440-07665-X

TO THOSE WHO LOVED SCOTT,
ESPECIALLY RONNIE AND STEVEN

Acknowledgments

I WISH to acknowledge my deepest thanks and appreciation to Miss Mary Ames Anderson, former Director of Public Relations of Childrens Hospital of Los Angeles and author, who first recognized the value of what Scott had to say to those who work with ill children; Mr. Darryl Ponicsan, author, who recognized Scott's talent and who said that his story should be told; and Miss Harriet Weaver, teacher, friend, and author, who told me that I was the one who should finish telling Scott's story. Mary Anderson, Darryl Ponicsan, and Harriet Weaver, all talented authors, acted on blind faith and gave me their wholehearted support and encouragement, helping me through the dark moments of this book.

I acknowledge with love and appreciation all the personnel of Childrens Hospital of Los Angeles, especially Dr. Kenneth Williams, who gave Scott a few more precious years to be with us.

Special thanks to my sister, Phyllis McMaster, for the hours she spent helping me type this book.

Foreword

THE MEMORY of Scott is surrounded with the military and bravery and medals. His short life revolved around dreams of heroes and heroic deeds. The physical battle as well as the result or the cause of the war. He was well beyond his time in his thinking.

He literally knew about the things men did in battle. He knew the loneliness of combat. The pain of the wound. The confidence of victory. The fear of defeat. The pride of valor. The modesty of spirit.

You could no more describe Scott's philosophy than you could tell what was going on in the minds of men in combat. You would have to know the person. You'd have to be there.

Scott's is not a story of a little boy who was sick. His is a story of a kid with guts and pride. Who was polite and tolerant. He spent most of his life with sophisticated people and played with children of his age and did the things young boys do.

But somehow he lived quite an adult existence of reality and decisions usually reserved for those of more advanced years. Or, sometimes, those thrown into situations requiring more mature reasoning.

I'm glad he got to do some of the things he had dreamed of.

I wasn't at all surprised to see him cope with the adult situations and wrestle with some of the problems . . . and hold his own. But I never ceased to be amazed at his knowledge and tolerance.

When Scott would call me on the telephone, he'd say, "Hello . . . this is Scott." Calmly. Precise. Exact. No commander on the field of battle ever summed it up and said it any better.

"Hello . . . this is Scott!"

Webb McKelvey,
Scott's friend

Publisher's Foreword

Wᴇ ɴᴇᴠᴇʀ knew Scott Ipswitch. But after reading his mother's manuscript, we felt as if we had known him well. A merry boy, sensitive and loving, intelligent, courageous. Very courageous.

Scott was fifteen when he died. For a third of his life he had fought Hodgkin's disease, a cancer that affects the lymph system. Fought so hard that he lived almost three years longer than the doctors thought possible. Fought even when his body was wasted and his vitality ebbing.

"There is barely any strength left in my body or soul to fight the battle I must fight," he wrote during the last weeks of his life. "I am so tired. I want just a little rest. But no. I must hurry. The fight continues without pause. I will conquer or die."

Scott never gave up. And he rarely complained. In his secret green notebook, which his parents read only after his death, Scott wrote, "If I would scream, venting my frustration through my scarred, pneumonia-filled, dilapidated lungs, the mountains would tremble, the creeks stop flowing. The summer air would frost. The trees would shed their leaves. And the land would weep." But all Scott's screams were silent.

He desperately wanted to live. "I must accomplish something. I must live a little longer, experience a little more. I must think. I *must* live. I want to."

Scott did accomplish something. His writings about his disease and his emotions have a poetic clarity that stirs the reader. They have been presented at medical and psychiatric conferences in this country and abroad. One doctor, tears in her eyes, said, "I hope I'll never be so tired that I'll forget I'm treating a human being," after reading Scott's manuscript.

Scott's story is not a sad story. It is an inspiring celebration of the human spirit. We feel privileged that Elaine Ipswitch has shared her son's story with us. We feel enriched because Scott was here.

Chapter One

I FOUND another one this morning.

I was out back moving things around to make room for the fall stock when I spotted it.

And I laughed. Out loud.

If anyone had told me last year that I would laugh over Scott, I would not have believed it. I would probably have burst into tears at the very idea. But this morning I laughed. On the wall where it had been hidden behind shoe boxes was a tiny drawing of a mouse, hardly larger than my thumbnail. An alert little mouse. His whiskers almost aquiver. Beside it in the small, precise hand I know so well was, "Scott was here."

Scott *was* here. And he will always be here in our hearts.

We had been a happy family, Ronnie and I and our twin sons, Steven and Scott. Ronnie and I had both grown up here in Fillmore, California. It was and still is a small town, a place of streets lined with palm trees, of avocado and walnut and orange groves nestled in a protecting ring of mountains that screen us from the Los Angeles smog.

After we got married, we lived in Los Angeles where

Ronnie worked for the telephone company, then after the boys were born, we moved to Ventura, a thirty-minute drive from Fillmore, and Ronnie worked as a lineman for Southern California Edison. Later on when Ronnie's folks, who owned the Fillmore Bootery, decided that they wanted to take life a bit easier, they offered Ronnie a partnership in the business and we moved back to Fillmore.

One of the benefits was that I could work part time in the store and see more of Ronnie. I felt right at home in the Fillmore Bootery. My father and mother had owned a small grocery store and meat market in Fillmore, and my sister Phyllis and I had both helped out after school. I had started working in the grocery when I was fourteen, which was when Ronnie and I first began to date. Ronnie and I both knew what it was like to be behind a counter and wait on customers, and I think this created an extra-strong bond between us. At any rate, we decided that when our boys were fourteen we would expect them to work just as we had. We wanted them to have the same sense of independence that we had enjoyed in our high school years.

About the time Ronnie and I got married, my parents sold their business and moved to Ventura where Phyllis and her children, Mark and Kym, were then living. But living in Ventura was just not the same as living in Fillmore. And eventually my parents and my sister and her family moved back, just as Ronnie and I had. Fillmore is a very special place.

Scott and Steven were nine at the time, excited at the prospect of hiking and fishing in the rugged mountains that began practically at the end of our street. We allowed ourselves one big luxury, a swimming pool in the backyard. Ronnie did a lot of the work himself and the boys helped. It became a gathering place for our family and friends. In the evenings Ronnie and I liked to sit beside the pool watching the afterglow of the sunset reflected on the low mountains until the sky darkened and the stars began to appear and it was time to tuck Scott and Steven in bed and kiss them good night.

It was a good life and a quiet one, although we were shaken up occasionally. Literally. Fillmore is on the rim of what geologists call the San Cayetano Thrust Fault. San Cayetano is the largest of the mountains that bulk above the town. The fault, I have been told, is related to the San Andreas Fault that runs the length of California. Every once in a while, there is a tremor, a shudder that rattles the dishes on the shelves and sets the mockingbirds to fussing. One tremor loosened and broke some of the blue border tiles of the swimming pool. Another spread a threatening web of cracks across a corner of the patio. Sometimes it is more than a shudder. I remember when I was a little girl waking up because my bed was shaking so hard. One early morning just after we moved back to Fillmore, there was a really big earthquake, so strong that Scott was thrown against the wall as he and Steven ran down the hall to our room.

Ronnie and I have taken the fragility of the earth's crust for granted all our lives. We never suspected that our happiness, which was solidly based on our love for each other and for our sons, was far more fragile, more susceptible to destruction than the china on our shelves. The first crack in our happiness appeared about a year after we had moved back to Fillmore.

The boys were ten, incredibly active and vital. In late August they had tried out for the Fillmore Youth Football Team and had been able to keep up with the bigger boys. They had passed their physical, but were too light to make the team. Scott weighed 54½ pounds and Steven, 53. The minimum weight for the team was 55 pounds.

I hoped this disappointment would motivate them to eat more. They were both picky eaters. But it did not. In fact I noticed toward the end of September that Scott was eating less than usual. His appetite stayed poor for a couple of weeks, and we began to crack down on him. At night when Scott just pushed the food around on his plate, Ronnie would tell him to stop fooling around and eat. Scott would say that he couldn't. And I would say, "Yes, you can. There's no reason why you can't." Then Scott began to say that he had a sore throat and it hurt to swallow. We thought this was just another one of his excuses. His throat was not red. He did not have a temperature. We just kept on getting cross with him. Finally Ronnie, exasperated, said, "Okay, you're going to go see Dr. Boatwright and find out why you can't swallow. And there'd better be a good reason."

The next day Dr. Boatwright peered down Scott's throat and found nothing. He said that often a throat could be terribly sore even if there was no inflammation and gave us a prescription for an antibiotic. "If it doesn't get better, come back in a week," he told us.

It did not get better. Scott started carrying a paper cup around with him to spit in because he could not swallow his saliva. He was eating next to nothing. Whenever I nagged at him to eat, he just shook his head and said, "Mom, it hurts to swallow."

Finally I asked, "Just where does it hurt?"

"Here," he said, and pointed not at his throat but several inches below in the area of his sternum.

We went back to Dr. Boatwright. I told him that Scott was no better. He got out his pad and started to write another prescription. "Dr. Boatwright," I said, "it is something more than just a sore throat. Scott, show him where it hurts to swallow."

Scott pointed to his sternum again. Dr. Boatwright nodded. "Well, perhaps you should see a throat specialist," he said. He recommended Dr. Blodget. Phil Blodget had been a few years ahead of Ronnie and me at Fillmore High School. He had had Hodgkin's disease in medical school and we had all been worried about him, but he was fine now. I made an appointment for Scott to see him the very next day, Thursday.

Dr. Blodget sent us to the hospital for X rays. "He may have some small object lodged in his throat," he told me, "or perhaps some glands are swollen and pressing against his esophagus. The X rays will show us which it is." I drove Scott straight to the hospital. They took X rays, then a second set, then a third. I drove back to Dr. Blodget's. He was grave as he asked me to come into his office.

"Elaine, the X rays show swollen glands and spots on Scott's lung," he said gently. He suggested that I take Scott to Dr. Martin, a pediatrician in Ventura, for tests. "If he can't see you right away, call me," he said, "and I'll talk to him."

I thanked him and got up to leave. Then I stopped. "You said spots on his lung?" I asked.

"Yes."

Dr. Martin was busy. He could not see Scott that afternoon, but he would make time for us first thing in the morning. I drove home slowly. Beside me, Scott was choking and coughing and spitting into his paper cup every few minutes.

Ronnie and I talked late into the night. We decided Scott must have tuberculosis. Those spots on his lung. His lack of appetite. They fit the description in our home medical guide. We would fix up our bedroom, which had its own bathroom, so Scott could recover at home and not have to go to a hospital. Discussing practical details made us feel better.

Then, Friday morning after Dr. Martin examined Scott, he led me into his office and closed the door. "I'm afraid Scott's got real problems," he said. "The X rays show swollen glands. Here and here." He pointed on the X ray. "And spots on his lungs. Here and here."

"Not both lungs!" I protested, panicked.

"These can be caused by a number of things," Dr. Martin went on, "tuberculosis, valley fever, virus infections, tumors. I tell you what. I'd like to run some blood tests and do some more X rays today, then on Monday I'd like to put Scott in the hospital for a few days so we can run more tests." With every word he said, I was getting more frightened. My eyes filled with tears. Dr. Martin looked at me closely, then he asked, "Would you feel better if we hospitalized Scott right now? We could get the test results that much sooner."

I nodded.

We returned to the examining room where Scott was waiting for us. Sitting on the examining table, his legs dangling, he looked very small and vulnerable. He was still a little boy. Just ten. But a strong, healthy little boy. Tan with sun-bleached hair, a wide, sweet smile, and big, trusting brown eyes. How could it be that we were suddenly talking of tuberculosis and tumors in connection with this sturdy son of mine? But was he so sturdy? He had lost weight the last few weeks. And he did seem pale under his tan. A shiver ran down my back.

"Well, Scott, I think we're going to put you in the hospital for a few days," Dr. Martin told him. "We'll do some tests and see if we can find out what is causing your problem."

Scott's face changed. He looked scared, almost as if he were lost. The last thing he could have expected to hear was that he was going to have to go to the hospital. And for what? No one knew.

If we were at all different from other happy families, it was because we considered our sons perhaps even more precious than most parents do. We had almost lost them.

When I was pregnant, we had not expected twins. In all the months of waiting and checkups, the obstetrician had only felt one head, only heard one heartbeat. But one very early morning in January 1961, six weeks ahead of time, I gave birth to Steven and three minutes later to Scott. They were identical tiny babies. Steven weighed only three pounds four ounces; Scott, four pounds six ounces.

Later I learned that this was not unusual. About half of all twin births are not discovered until delivery. But, you can imagine our surprise at the time.

Shortly after I was wheeled back to my room, the doctor came to see me. "Don't get your hopes up," he said. "They're very small and very frail." They had only a twenty-five percent chance of living, he warned me.

As soon as they were born, they had been rushed into the premature ward where they could be monitored constantly. I had to look at them through a window. The thought that we might lose them without my ever having held them in my arms was agonizing. Scott slowly grew stronger and graduated from the premature ward to a crib in the nursery. One day they allowed me to put on a gown and mask and stand next to his crib. It was the first time since he was born that I had seen him close up. I reached out to touch his foot—it was unbelievably tiny—but the nurse caught my hand. "I'm sorry," she said, "you're not allowed to touch him." I tried to understand but it was very hard. Scott finally came home when he was two weeks old, but Steven went through crisis after crisis. His weight dropped to two and a half pounds. He was three months old before he was strong enough to come home.

Because of those frightening early days, we had never been able to take our boys for granted. We treasured them. And we delighted in them. Even in their mischief. Even though they were identical twins, we made a point of calling them the boys rather than the twins, and I did not dress them alike. We wanted them to be individuals. But they soon learned how to take advantage of being twins.

One morning when they were about two, Steven came in from the backyard and asked for a cookie. "I just gave you one," I said.

"No, that was Scott," he said.

"I know who you are, Steven. One is all you get." And he laughed and ran out again.

They used to beg me to read aloud to them. Their first day in kindergarten was a sharp disappointment. They had been sure they were going to learn how to read and that they would be able to read the newspaper that very night with their daddy. They felt cheated. But it was not long before they were reading and writing. My sister gave them a double desk and chairs and they used to spend hours at it drawing pictures and writing stories. So, later on, it was natural for Scott to write about his medical experiences. He wrote about everything.

> The date is October 29, 1971. After several weeks of complaining of trouble with swallowing, Mom took me to Dr. Boatwright, Dr. Blodget and Dr. Martin. Dr. Martin asked me if I would mind going into the hospital for a few days. He said I would probably miss Hallowe'en. I said I wouldn't mind. I knew something was wrong with my health.
>
> I walk into the hospital, into a room. I get into some stupid looking pajamas. I was in bed and I was a bit scared. A doctor came in and poked at my neck, stomach and other places. Then he took a syringe full of my blood.

All afternoon technicians kept coming in to draw blood for the tests that Dr. Martin had ordered. "Why can't they take all the blood they need at one time," Scott asked, "instead of coming in and sticking me every five minutes?"

"There's a reason," Dr. Martin explained. "The technicians mix the blood with different chemical solutions for different tests. For some they have to have fresh blood straight from your vein. For others, the blood has to stand for several hours, sometimes for a few days, for blood cultures before they do the tests."

Scott began counting the needle "sticks." He had reached 117 when he stopped keeping track a few days before he left the hospital.

Scott's roommate had been in the hospital for seven months. Monty had been riding on an oil pump, the kind that looks like a horse. He slipped and was crushed by the metal arm. "We were afraid he would die," his mother told me, "but he's going to make it. Monty had had several operations already and faced more surgery and painful skin grafts.

"How do you stand it?" I asked her.

"I just think of what Monty has gone through and is still going through," she said. "He's the one who is in pain. I try to be as strong as I can for his sake."

When visiting hours were over that day, Dr. Martin walked down the hall with Ronnie and me. He said he was ordering more tests, including skin tests to see whether Scott's problems might be caused by some virus or fungous infection. And then he looked straight at me. "Elaine, you can cry all you want on the inside. But not on the outside. Remember, Scott looks to you for courage." It was Scott's first day in the hospital and I was learning my first lesson. I must conceal my pain. I must be brave for Scott. I tried hard. But Scott did far better than I did.

When everybody left, I just lay there in bed feeling a bit worried and grey. I didn't get much sleep that night. Babies crying! Trays rattling! Shoes clicking on the floor! Moans! I could hardly stand it!

In the morning, I heard rattling. A tray appeared filled with needles, syringes, test tubes and things. They drew some blood from me. Then they went away and I had breakfast. The day was filled with tests. A doctor came in with this machine. It had a mask and he put it over my nose and mouth. It was salt air and when I breathed it, I would cough. He wanted me to cough up stuff from way down in my lungs. For hours I was breathing that salt-filled air. I was nearly coughing to death. After what seemed an eternity, they went away. But without a drop of stuff from my lungs.

Needles, shots, injections and a few unmentionable items tested me constantly. Doctors seemed to get a kick out of feeling, peering and poking at me. I kept asking what was the matter with me and the doctors would just say "That's what we're trying to find out."

Scott's arms were beginning to look interesting, to say the least, with the skin-patch tests, each identified by a painted circle or square or triangle, the needle marks, and the bruises from the blood tests. His veins were hard to find and hit. As the days went by it was harder and harder for the technicians to hit a vein on the first try. It got so that when they came in, Scott would just moan, "Oh, no."

When Ronnie and I talked with Dr. Martin on Sunday, all he had to report was no progress. "Nothing's shown up yet in the tests. One of the men in the lab is certain Scott has some type of infection. The others are not so sure," he said. "We have to wait a few days for the rest of the tests to be completed."

> The third day a doctor told me I was going to have a bone marrow. He explained everything about it to me. He had one done on him in medical school. There had not been anything wrong with him. It was just that the med students wanted to practice. He said it hurt pretty bad.
>
> About seven people gathered around my bed. There was a doctor, a couple of residents, nurses and technicians. The doctor asked me if I was ready. I felt a few people's hands clamp down over me. The doctor worked that big needle in my sternum and I lurched a bit. My mouth opened and I lay there completely still and let out a long silent scream that no one heard but me.

The doctor had told me it might be hard for me to watch the bone-marrow test and suggested that I wait outside. I asked Scott what he would like. "I'd like you to stay and hold my hand," he said. And I did.

It is a grim procedure. Scott was given Novocaine injections, but the doctor explained that since the anesthetic could not penetrate bone, it would hurt when the needle hit and entered the bone. They push a hollow needle, about a quarter of an inch in diameter, through the skin and into the bone. In Scott's case into his sternum. Once this large needle is in place, a smaller needle is inserted into it and right through into the bone cavity. Then the bone marrow is sucked up into the syringe.

After the test when everyone had left the room, Scott asked, "Mom, did I make too much noise?"

"Noise?" I said, surprised. "You didn't make a sound. I saw you open your mouth wide once, but you didn't say anything."

"Oh, I thought I screamed," he said.

Scott faced still more tests, all of them unpleasant, although perhaps not as cruel as the bone marrow. One night he had to drink castor oil before a series of X rays. He hated the stuff and it took almost an hour for him to get it down. The next day after he'd had his X rays, a nurse came in with another dose of castor oil. "I hate to have to tell you this," she said, "but the X rays showed some stool in your intestines, Scott. They have to do them over again tomorrow. You have to drink this now."

"I'm sure I'm empty now," he pleaded, but he had to drink it. That evening another nurse told him he had to have an enema. He had never had one before and did not like the idea at all. Nor its effects. He would exclaim, "Oh, Mom, my stomach hurts so!" and run toward the toilet time after time. I sat there by his bed, wondering just how much testing he could stand.

After every test we would hope that the doctors would now be able to tell us what was wrong, but the only real news during the first five days was that the bone-marrow test had been negative, which meant that he did not have leukemia. Finally when nothing showed up in the blood tests or the skin tests or the X rays, Dr. Martin said that the next step would be a bronchoscopy and a lymph node biopsy.

"Does that mean he has tumors?" I asked, not daring to say the word *cancer*.

"We don't know," he answered.

When Ronnie and I left Scott that night, we told him that we would be there when he woke up after his surgery the next day. It was hard to be cheerful and matter of fact. We were frightened. Really frightened. Maybe things were not going to "turn out all right" the way everyone kept telling us they would. But I could hope for one more night. I could hope that after the biopsy tomorrow the surgeon would say that the spots on Scott's lungs and the swollen glands were not caused by cancer. If he said that, then I could allow myself to break down and cry. In relief. In happiness. As we drove home, I kept imagining how good this would feel.

The doctor came in and told me what was going to happen. They would cut my neck, take out some lymph nodes and perform a bronchoscopy to find out what I had. A nurse came in and gave me a shot and told me to take off my pants.
"Why?" I asked.
"Just a rule we have in surgery," he said and wheeled me away to the operating room. There I was hooked up to machines, my neck was cleaned, an I.V. was started and I was given a shot that immediately put me to sleep.
I woke up in the recovery room. There were a lot of nurses. They kept giving me shots. Then I discovered myself in my room.

Ronnie and I had been at the hospital since early morning. It was a bright fall day, but the sunshine brought no cheer to the surgery waiting room. Somehow it seemed to make the waiting harder to bear. There was only one other person there, a woman whose eighteen-year-old son had been in a motorcycle accident the night before. "I hope this teaches him a lesson," she kept saying.

Dr. Martin came by at one point and told us that Scott was doing fine and would be out of surgery in about an hour. Almost two hours later, the surgeon walked into the waiting room. He was still wearing his operating greens.

"Scott is doing fine," he said. "He'll be in the recovery room for a while. Then he'll be taken back to his room."

"What does he have?" Ronnie asked. "Do you know yet?"

"Oh, yes. It's Hodgkin's. No doubt about it."

Chapter Two

"Scott has Hodgkin's disease," Dr. Martin confirmed the next day. "The biopsy shows it clearly. If the disease is confined to the area above his diaphragm, his chances are very good. If the area below is involved . . ." He hesitated, then went on: "Well, his chances are not so good."

Not so good? What does that mean? Not so good? I knew what it meant. And my heart plunged. Dr. Martin was still speaking. I had to force myself to pay attention. Ronnie was sitting there, tense, his eyes on the doctor's face.

"There are some decisions that must be made," Dr. Martin was saying, "as soon as possible."

"Today?" Ronnie asked. I remembered reading an article about the danger of making decisions when you are upset. How could we make decisions now? But it seemed that we had to.

"Now that we know Scott has Hodgkin's, we have to find out just what areas of his body are involved. This means more tests. And surgery."

Ronnie and I looked at each other. How many tests, how much surgery, how much pain could Scott bear? How much could we bear? But we knew the answers. We could bear anything, permit Scott to bear anything, if it would cure him. Still, we truly did not realize how much we would be asking Scott to bear.

"There are two ways we can handle this," Dr. Martin went on. "I can consult specialists at Childrens Hospital in Los Angeles, do the tests they order, and send the results to them for interpretation. They will decide what treatment Scott needs, and we can carry out the treatment here in Ventura.

"The alternative is to send Scott to Childrens Hospital."

We thought about this for a minute.

"What would you do if he were your son?" Ronnie asked.

"Send him to Childrens."

"Then that's what we'll do," Ronnie said.

Dr. Martin said he would make the arrangements. "We'll keep Scott here a few days to recover from the biopsy. Then depending on what they say at Childrens, he may be able to go home before going down there."

Hope seeped back. Scott would be coming home. The new tests would reveal that the disease had not invaded his body below the diaphragm. The doctors in Los Angeles would know how to cure him. God would not let Scott suffer.

I had been brought up as a Christian believing in God and in Jesus, believing what I read in the Bible. I truly believed that if you really wanted something, all you had to do was ask. If you were a Christian, you would get it. I had said my prayers every night since I was a little girl. After Scott and Steven were born, I always asked the Lord to please take care of my children. I never asked for a diamond or a big house. I just asked God to watch over my children.

As Ronnie and I were leaving the hospital that night,

we ran into a doctor who had gone to the same church we had when we lived in Ventura. We told him about the diagnosis and how worried we were.

"This is easier on us as believing Christians than on others," was his response. "Life is so short when compared to eternity." And he went on about how infinite eternity was. I listened in shock. He was talking as if Scott were going to die. I had been praying for Scott's recovery. I wanted to hear that God would heal him, not how long eternity was.

A couple of days later, our minister and his wife visited Scott in the hospital. Before I brought them in to see Scott, I had told them that he had Hodgkin's disease and that it could be very serious. "I can see that one day this will be all to God's glory," our minister said. I could not see that. How could it be to God's glory to let Scott die?

If I believed what I professed to believe, I should have agreed with these men. But suddenly my religious faith was being tested as it had never been before. I just could not make myself accept the idea that Scott's death was God's will.

Eleven days after Scott had unexpectedly been admitted to the hospital, I brought him home. He had lost weight and was white as a sheet, but he had a grin that lit up our house. That evening I looked around the room— my beloved husband, my beloved sons. I thought how you never appreciate how good your life is until disaster strikes. We were all so happy and thankful to be together. The telephone rang constantly. Our families, our friends, the boys' friends—they all wanted to know how Scott was and to tell him they were glad he was back home. When it rang during supper, I expected it to be just another "glad he's home" call. But it wasn't.

It was Dr. Martin. He had just heard from Childrens

Hospital. They wanted Scott there at one o'clock the next day.

It was a shock. Our laughter was stilled. We had counted so much on having a few days together. Scott needed to relax and build up his strength. Ronnie and I needed a respite from the fear that was growing inside us—like a cancer, I kept thinking. And Steven needed some reassurance and security. He was still a little boy and very bewildered by his brother's sudden illness. A few nights before at bedtime, he had told his grandmother that he felt as if he were in no-man's-land. When I heard this, I felt terrible. But I just didn't know what I could do. Scott needed me so much right now. I would have given anything to keep Scott at home for a few more days, but I knew the sooner the specialists at Childrens examined him and made their tests, the sooner they could start treating him. And the sooner he would get well.

Childrens Hospital seemed very large and frightening when Ronnie, Scott, and I walked in the next day at exactly one o'clock. We filled out forms and waited. We signed consent papers and waited. We were taken to the second floor where Scott gave a urine specimen and had a blood test and we waited some more. It was four o'clock before Scott was taken to a room on Four West (fourth floor, west wing, where most of the young patients were suffering from "catastrophic disease").

Ronnie and I had decided not to tell Scott that he had Hodgkin's. We cherished a wild hope that the new tests at Childrens would prove the original diagnosis mistaken. So when the nurse who filled out Scott's chart that first day called me over and pointed to the question that asked if the child knew what was wrong with him, I told him no. He wrote it down without comment.

It was after six when a tall, distinguished-looking man in a white coat strode into the room. "I'm Dr. Williams," he said and sat on the end of Scott's bed. "And you must be Scott." Dr. Kenneth Williams was the hematologist in charge of Scott's case. We liked him immediately. We had no idea then how important this gifted physician and very kind man would become in our lives.

He examined Scott and chatted with him a bit, asking about his brother and school. Then he said that he had scheduled a number of tests—blood tests (Scott groaned), more X rays, a lymphangiogram—and that they would start on them first thing in the morning. When Ronnie and I walked around the corner to the motel where we were staying that night, we agreed that we had done the right thing in bringing Scott down to Los Angeles. Dr. Williams inspired trust.

> It was scary to be having millions of tests every day and not even the doctors knowing what I had. The day came that I was to have my lymphangiogram. They inject blue dye between my toes, then make incisions on the tops of my feet and inject dye into my lymphatic tissue. Then they take x-rays of my lymphatic system with a special machine. The dye would show up on the x-rays, showing which lymph nodes and vessels were swollen. When I vomited or went to the bathroom, everything came out dark turquoise for the next few weeks. They got me ready for the operation by doping me all up. It is extremely painful.

Ronnie and I waited anxiously in Scott's room the morning of the lymphangiogram, which would show just how involved Scott's lymph system was. When the nurse rolled Scott back into the room after four hours, we were shocked to discover that he had not had the operation. The X-ray machine had been broken.

At the motel that night Ronnie and I asked each other why they hadn't checked the machine before preparing Scott for the operation. And if the machine was broken, why had they kept him lying on a stretcher outside sur-

gery all alone for all those hours? We were to ask ourselves a lot of questions like this. We asked ourselves,
because we were too scared to ask the nurses or the
doctors. They might get angry—and take it out on Scott.

> The next day they finally got the machine fixed. They
> started injecting the dye, which was very painful. I com-
> plained about them spilling the dye all over me. The
> nurse told me, "Just close your eyes and go to sleep."
>
> The doctor changed his surgical gloves about every
> minute because they would become drenched in blood. I
> couldn't believe that was my blood, my foot they were
> operating on. But it sure hurt.
>
> All of a sudden I woke up. I looked at my feet. They
> were wrapped in elastic bandages up to my knees. I
> thought they had crippled me. I started to cry.
>
> "What's the matter?" the assistant surgeon asked.
>
> "My feet," I sobbed. "What happened?" He patted
> me on the shoulder and smiled. "It'll be okay," he said.
> "Don't worry." Then they wheeled me out to the hall
> where I waited for about two hours. It was horrible. I
> was in pain and wanted to see Mom and Dad and ask
> them what had happened to my feet.

When they took Scott away this time, we were told the
operation would take about three hours. We started
worrying as the three hours stretched into four. And got
frightened when the nurse came in and asked where Scott
was, saying, "He should be back by now."

I went to the nurses' desk and asked if I could speak to
Dr. Gates, the intern who was involved with Scott's case.
No, she was in a meeting. How about Dr. Williams? No,
he was not available. I went back to wait some more.

Another nurse came in. "Isn't Scott back yet?"

"No, he's been gone five hours and we haven't heard a
thing."

"I'll go see what's taking so long," she said. In a few

minutes, she came back and said, "He should be here soon."

It was two hours later when they wheeled him back. Seven hours that Scott had been alone and in pain in a strange place. Later on, I learned that we could have been with him for at least four of those hours. But no one had thought to tell us.

Scott's days were punctuated by blood tests—five or six a day. After the first jab he would ask, "Did you get it?" It usually took a little probing to hit a vein. More and more often, the technician would withdraw the needle and say, "I'll have to try again." If the second try was successful, Scott would sigh with relief. If a third or fourth attempt was necessary, he turned his head away and the tears would roll silently down his face. The good spots were used over and over again until the vein collapsed. But the blood tests, no matter how painful, were truly pinpricks in comparison with what was to come.

One morning Dr. Williams told us it was time for Scott's staging operation. This was the crucial operation, the one that would tell us the extent of the disease, which stage it had reached.

There are four stages of Hodgkin's. In Stage One, the disease is limited to one region of the body. In Stage Two, it is in two or more regions of the body, but on only one side of the diaphragm. Dr. Martin had told us that if Scott's Hodgkin's was confined to the area above his diaphragm, he would have a pretty good chance of recovery. In Stage Three, the disease is on both sides of the diaphragm, involving only the lymph nodes and spleen and in Stage Four, the disease has disseminated beyond Stage Three to diffusely involve the lung, liver, bone marrow, skin or central nervous system. Each stage is divided into A and B, depending on whether the victim has fever or night sweats or significant weight loss.

When Dr. Williams introduced us to Dr. Morton Woolley, who was going to perform the staging operation, the surgeon asked us if we had any questions. Ronnie and I were silent. We could not think of anything. "I guess not," I answered finally. A couple of seconds later, I ran down the corridor after Dr. Woolley. "Scott is so thin and weak. Isn't it dangerous to operate now?" I asked.

"There's always a risk in surgery," he said, "but Scott's not getting any better. We need to know the results of tests that can only be made if we operate, if we are going to help him."

"It has to be done?"

"It has to be done." Then he smiled and said, "I think he'll come through it fine."

I was wheeled into the surgery waiting room. The surgeons were at a desk, talking and looking at x-rays. Someone wheeled me through some doors. I started praying. They moved me onto a cold, green table. Three big lights peered at me. For quite a while they were taping things to me. I would ask them about the machines and they would tell me about them. Then they started swabbing me with antiseptic. COLD! How COLD that stuff is! Then he put the mask on me and let me hold it on. The lights started spinning. Slow, then a little faster, faster . . . spin, spin, spin!

"STOP!" I shouted. I wanted the lights to stop spinning. I could hear the surgeons talking. Their faces jumped into the light. All I could see were the lights spinning and the surgeons' faces spinning in them. The anesthesiologist was talking to me, telling me, "It will be all right. Just try to sleep."

"Stop it! Please, stop it! Let me out!" I cried. I couldn't see any more. All I could do was hear them talk.

I opened my eyes. I saw Mom. I tried to make a

sound. I hurt all over. I hurt where the tubes were stuck in me. My gut hurt. It hurt to breathe. I was thirsty. I closed my eyes and went back to sleep. I opened my eyes again. Mom held my hand. She told me that Dr. Woolley had said that everything went well. I still hurt. I fell asleep again.

My surgery consisted of a splenectomy, appendectomy, multiple lymph node biopsies, a liver biopsy, a bone biopsy and a bronchoscopy. It was a major operation. There were 30 stitches in the incision that went from my last rib down to my groin and five stitches in my hip where they took out a piece of bone.

Dr. Williams led Ronnie and me to a conference room down the hall from Scott's room. Dr. Gates, the intern, and Dr. Barak, a hematology fellow who was involved with Scott's case, were with him. The doctors sat on one side of the long table, Ronnie and I on the other. I could find no sign of hope in those three serious faces across from us.

Dr. Williams opened his folder. "Scott's spleen was grossly enlarged and involved with Hodgkin's disease," he reported. "The lymph node biopsies were positive, showing involvement of the nodes both above and below the diaphragm. His lungs are involved. The bone biopsy was negative. It will be a few days before we have the liver biopsy results."

He paused.

"We have classified Scott's disease at Stage Four B," he said quietly.

It could not have been worse.

After a moment he went on: "Scott's case will be presented at the next Tumor Board and his course of treatment will be determined then. Do you have any questions?"

Don't cry, I told myself. Think. What do I need to

know? I could think of only one thing. "How long does someone [I could not use Scott's name] live when he has Stage Four Hodgkin's?"

"About two years," Dr. Williams said.

There was a gasp next to me. Ronnie was holding his head in his hands. Then there was silence. After a few minutes, the three doctors got up. The door closed behind them.

Ronnie walked over to the window. He hit the wall. "No, I don't believe it!" We held on to each other. We were drowning in sorrow—for Scott, for ourselves. "I don't want him to know," Ronnie said. "We'll tell him he's going to be fine. We'll keep this a secret between us. I don't want anyone to know he's going to die."

This decision helped. It gave us the illusion of being in control. We were able to go back to Scott's room and tell him without breaking down. As soon as we walked in, he asked, "Do they know what I've got?"

Very matter-of-factly I said, "They just told us that you've got Hodgkin's disease."

"Is it curable?"

"Oh, yes," I reassured him. "Do you remember Dr. Blodget? He had Hodgkin's when he was in medical school."

"Dr. Blodget had this?"

"That's right." I was glad Scott had seen Dr. Blodget. I thought I might ask him to talk to Scott later on. "The doctors are going to have a special meeting to decide just how they are going to treat you to cure it."

Scott said, "Oh."

And that was all.

We did not tell him that Hodgkin's was a form of cancer. If we had told Scott that Hodgkin's was cancer, that is about all we would have been able to tell him. We knew so little about the disease. Later that day I stopped

Dr. Gates in the hall and asked the question that was tormenting me: "How does a person die from Hodgkin's?"

"From an infection usually," she told me. "Like pneumonia. Their lymph system can't fight the infection." I did not understand then that she was telling me that Scott's death could be merciful and quick.

Even though I had asked the question, I was resisting the knowledge that Hodgkin's could kill. "We know people who had Hodgkin's who have been cured," I insisted. There were several people in Fillmore who had had the disease. I realized later that I had no idea what stage their Hodgkin's had been. The cure rate for adults with Stage One is around eighty percent.

"It does happen," Dr. Gates said. "And there are cases where spontaneous remissions have occurred."

"We'll hope for a spontaneous remission for Scott," I said firmly.

She smiled. "You should never give up hope," she said and gave me a quick hug. I asked her if she could recommend something that I could read about Hodgkin's. She shook her head. "There's some material in my medical textbooks, but it's all so technical I don't think you'd get anything out of it."

The next day Ronnie asked one of the doctors, "What can you tell us about Hodgkin's?" I will never forget that doctor sitting there and saying, "Well, I'm trying to think how I can bring it down to a level that you will understand." Later Ronnie said, "I felt like telling him, you just talk to me on your level. I'll ask questions if I don't understand."

When we asked Dr. Williams what we could read to learn about Hodgkin's, he told us that the only meaningful information was in medical journals, but that by the time it was published, it was already obsolete because such strides were being made in treatment. He also told us that childhood Hodgkin's was so rare that very little had been written about it. It usually attacks people between twenty and thirty and over fifty.

Dr. Williams explained that it was a cancer of the lymphatic system. And that the lymphatic system is the network of nodes or glands and vessels that manufacture and circulate lymphocytes and plasma cells through the body to fight infections.

We learned that the disease was named after Thomas Hodgkin, an English physician who has been described as being a century ahead of his time—that time being the early nineteenth century. His paper, "On Some Morbid Appearances of the Absorbent Glands and Spleen," which he presented before the Medical-Chirurgical Society of London in 1832, was the first description of the disease. And we learned that Dorothy Reed's description in 1902 of the cells, now known as Reed-Sternberg cells, found in the lymph nodes of people who have Hodgkin's, first made positive diagnosis possible. And that it was not until after World War Two that significant advances were made in treatment, radiotherapy, and especially chemotherapy benefiting from wartime research.

But we wanted to know more. We wanted to know what to expect. What we could hope for. And no one would—or could—tell us these things. Doctors are still learning about Hodgkin's disease. They learned from Scott, and so did we as the years went by.

The first sign of Hodgkin's is usually (but not always) a swollen gland in the neck, which may not even be noticed until it is large enough to exert pressure or produce obstructive symptoms. This is what happened with Scott, who had no symptoms until he began having trouble swallowing.

Hospital life was strange—and sometimes cruel. Scott still had trouble swallowing and his appetite was even poorer after the staging operation. Every mouthful of food he got down represented a triumph for him. The nurses understood this. They left his tray with him for a long time. They encouraged him to try to eat and never hurried him. But a couple of times a week student nurses took over from the regular nurses—changing beds, giving baths, and helping with the meals. One of them gave Scott his lunch one day. When she came back, he had barely touched his food.

"Scott, aren't you going to eat your lunch?" she asked.

"Yes," he said, "but it takes me a little while because it hurts to swallow." And he pushed the food around his plate a little, took a few bites, drank a little milk, and said he was finished.

"You have to eat more than that," the student told him.

"I can't."

"Come on, try."

"I can't," Scott said emphatically.

"What's the matter? Don't you want to get well?"

That did it. "Yes," Scott yelled, "I want to get well, but it hurts to swallow. That's why I'm here. Why can't anyone seem to understand that?" And he started crying.

I had been staying out of this, hoping that the nurse might coax Scott to eat more, but her last remark was so innocently cruel that I could not stand it and I rushed out of the room. The nurse at the desk looked up and saw that I was crying. I told her what had happened and said that I just had to go to the rest room until I could pull myself together.

"Why don't you go to the parents' room?" she asked.

"Parents' room?"

And she showed me a room down the hall that I had never known existed. It had a sofa, chairs, television set, and its own toilet and washbasin. I locked myself inside and cried until there were no more tears. And then I looked around, wondering why no one had told me about it before. I learned later that it was called the crying room.

When I went back to Scott, he asked if I had left because I was angry with him. I explained that I was just upset at what the student nurse had said to him, that I knew he tried hard to eat and get strong. "The nurse was trying to help," I said, "even though she went about it the wrong way." And then I sighed. "Scott, I love you so much. I wish I could take all this pain from you."

"If I could give it to you, Mom, I wouldn't," he said.

"I'd make you," I told him with a smile.

"No," he said seriously, "I'd never want you to go through this."

A long time afterward when he was home again and feeling well, I asked him what he was thinking those days in the hospital after his surgery.

"I thought I was dying," he said.

"Oh, Scott," I exclaimed, "I'm so sorry. Why didn't you tell me?" And yet, as I said it, I was glad that he had not. I wouldn't have known what to say to him.

> **One night I had a dream. My dog Trampas was sitting on my bed. I called for him, but he disappeared. I stared at where I had seen him. It shattered me into a billion pieces. Tears welled up in my eyes and all I wanted was to go home.**

Home seemed very far away. Both Scott and I began to think that just being home would solve everything. The nights in the hospital were the hardest. During the day, nurses and technicians would be coming and going, drawing blood, taking temperatures, giving baths, the whole hospital routine. But the evenings, especially when Ron-

nie was not able to drive down from Fillmore and there
were no other visitors, were long and sad.

I used to wheel Scott around Four West to give him a
change of scenery. We always spent ten or fifteen minutes
watching the fish in the aquarium at the nurses' station.
One night a nurse asked if we had been to the penthouse
and told us how to get there. We went up and found
ourselves in a corridor with huge windows on both sides
and the lights of Los Angeles stretched out below us.
Outside on the roof was a helicopter pad. Scott always
hoped we'd see a helicopter settle down on it, but we
never did.

The penthouse became a haven. It was quiet after Four
West, where the television sets were on constantly and
children were crying and running around. Scott could
not see very well from his wheelchair, so I would lift him
up so he could look out over the city with me. I would
think about all the thousands of people out there leading
normal lives and wish that we could go back to the way
we had been before. I would wonder what I would do if
Scott died. There were times when I was so upset that I
thought I'd just sneak his body out of the hospital and
run away with him. Nobody would take him from me.
Ever. Other times I thought I would jump from the
penthouse roof, but this was just melodrama. I could
never leave Ronnie and Steven. But those were the
thoughts that went through my mind.

When I said I felt terribly burdened, a friend suggested
that I read the Book of Job. So one night at a nearby
motel where I was staying for a while I picked up the
Gideon Bible and read the Book of Job. And then I was
really frightened, more emotionally upset than ever. Job
"saw his sons, and his sons' sons, even four generations,"
but those first sons who had been killed by the great wind
from the wilderness were lost to him forever. I did not

want Scott to be lost to me forever. But I found something else in the Bible that did help me, a verse from
Hebrews: "Now faith is the substance of things hoped
for, the evidence of things not seen." And I told myself
this had to be my answer for now.

The next night when I left Scott to go to the motel, he
asked me to stay because he was scared. I said I'd stay a
little longer, but I couldn't stay all night because I
needed to get some sleep. "Scott, whenever you're scared,"
I told him, "and I'm not here to talk to, you can talk to
God, you know. Say a prayer. He'll listen." And I was
sure He would listen to Scott, even if He didn't seem to
be listening to me.

"Mom, I haven't stopped praying since the day I came
here," he answered.

When the Tumor Board at Childrens discussed Scott's
case after the staging operation, they decided he should
be treated by chemotherapy. Most cases are treated by
radiotherapy or a combination of radiation and chemotherapy, but Scott's body was so riddled with Hodgkin's
that Dr. Williams said that if they were to attempt to kill
the cancer cells with radiation, they would kill Scott in
the process.

He said that the drugs they would be using had already
been used with some success at the Stanford Medical
Center in Palo Alto. This was enough to start me hoping
again. "Scott will be getting three drugs a day in pill
form," he said, "and two intravenously at weekly intervals. We're going to start the treatment tomorrow."

At last. After all these weeks and all the tests and surgery, they were ready to attack the disease.

Cytoxan, vincristine, Matulane, prednisone, isoniazid.
I read the names of the drugs on the consent form and
signed it. A few minutes later I could not remember the

names of the drugs or even which would be given when. But I got to know them well. They were harsh drugs with harsh side effects. Their mission was to destroy the cancer cells, but they attacked healthy cells as well. It was up to the doctors to find the therapeutic balance.

Scott had to take twelve pills a day. It seemed as if the medicine nurse was always popping into his room. After a couple of days, Scott started complaining. It still hurt to swallow. How could we expect him to get all those pills down, in addition to the liquid medicine he was getting to break up the congestion in his lungs. And the pills tasted bad. He was so slow taking them that the medicine nurse began leaving them with me after I promised that I would see to it that Scott got every last one of them down.

And then he really started. He would take out all his frustrations on me. He would cry that he just couldn't swallow. He would shout and say I should know by now that he couldn't swallow. And I did know. But neither his crying nor his shouting weakened my resolve. He had to swallow those pills. And he did. I was going to see to it that he got well—no matter how unpleasant the process.

And it was unpleasant. All of it. On the day Scott was finally discharged from Childrens, he had his second intravenous chemotherapy treatment, and Ronnie and I had a briefing from Dr. Barak, the hematology fellow, on the effects of these treatments. He explained that Scott would probably vomit for a few hours or even a few days after each treatment. "And he may start to lose his hair. Some children lose all their hair," Dr. Barak said. "With others it seems to fall out in patches." I had noticed that a number of the children on Four West wore hats all the time to hide their bald heads.

"We can't tell now just how the drugs will affect his growth," he said. "We'll just have to wait and see. Another side effect is that the drugs cause a decrease in the

white cells. This means that Scott will be more susceptible to colds and infections."

"What about school?" I asked. "Should we keep him
home so that he won't be exposed to the other children's
colds and germs?"

"Absolutely not. He should go back to school as soon as
he's strong enough," Dr. Barak said emphatically. "It's
important for him to lead a normal life. We can handle
colds and many infections with antibiotics. Just be careful. And don't worry too much."

"He's right," Ronnie said. "We can't keep him
wrapped in cotton wool. That would be cruel."

Finally we were ready to leave. These had been the
three longest weeks in our lives. As Scott said, it seemed
as if he had been in the hospital "forever." Scott was
dressed and Ronnie had gone to get the car when Dr.
Gates came to say good-bye. As she was leaving, she put
her hand to her forehead. "Dr. Williams asked me to tell
you something. What in the world was it? For the life of
me, I can't remember."

I thought I knew. I was sure he had asked her to tell us
the results of Scott's liver biopsy. It had been two weeks
since Dr. Williams had reported the findings of the staging operation and said that it would be a few days before
they would have the results of the liver biopsy. I started
to ask Dr. Gates if that was what he had asked her to tell
us, but I stopped. I had a feeling I knew the answer—and
I did not want to hear it. Just a few weeks earlier, I had
wanted to know the results of each test as soon as possible.
But I had been full of hope then. My only hope now was
that perhaps the Hodgkin's had not spread to Scott's
liver. I needed to hold on to that hope a little longer.

"You'll think of it," I told her. "You can call us later
and tell us." And five minutes later, Scott and I walked

out of the hospital and got into the car with Ronnie to go home.

It was November 30. From now on Scott would be an outpatient seeing Dr. Williams at the Hematology-Oncology Clinic at Childrens. His first appointment was scheduled for two days after Christmas.

I remember the ride home. I saw the bare walnut trees as we neared Fillmore. They had been green the last time I saw them. It was sunset—and a beautiful one—as we drove by the trees, the river. I saw birds, rocks, bushes, grass, water. For more than a month I had not been outside. I had not seen a bit of greenery except for hospital flowers. It was so wonderful. The trees, grass, birds, even the sun seemed to greet me. So I said hello back to them.

I snuggled into my very own bed for the first time in a month. And for the first time in way over a month, I was really truly happy.

Chapter Three

ALL these weeks I had felt as if I were sliding down a chute in the dark, not knowing where I was or where I was going. Simply aware that there was no turning back. Now I had arrived. At a way station admittedly, not the final destination. The medical verdict could not have been worse, but in a curious way, having the diagnosis confirmed provided a respite. We were no longer in limbo. It was time to explore where we were—Scott and Steve and Ronnie and I. Nothing would ever be the same again. So much in our lives had changed.

Scott's illness was taking its toll of all of us—a physical and emotional toll. Not, surprisingly enough, a financial one. We had expected that the medical expenses would wipe us out. We had no medical insurance. When Ronnie left Southern California Edison, we had dropped Blue Cross, because we could not afford the hundred-dollar-a-month individual rate. If there were medical emergencies, we decided at that time, we would just have to borrow money or see if we could make monthly payments.

Now we worried that if we could not pay Scott's medical bills, they might be collected against the store and destroy the business that Ronnie's parents, Jack and

Roma, had spent nearly twenty years building. Ronnie and I consulted a lawyer about dissolving the partnership with his parents, but he advised us that we could be accused of fraud if it were shown that we had dissolved the partnership after learning that we were going to incur huge medical bills.

When Dr. Martin learned that we had no insurance, he made an appointment for us with Crippled Children's Services, a program set up by the California State Department of Health and financed by federal, state, and county tax funds to help families of children who have catastrophic diseases.

We were pretty discouraged when we went to CCS. All we knew was that Scott had to get the best care available and we had to pay for it. Somehow. No matter what. We figured that we were young enough so each of us could work at two jobs. And we'd just have to borrow the rest of the money. But CCS explained that its interest was in seeing that families were able to survive, in seeing that parents did not have to work at two jobs and neglect both their ill and their well children. They were not interested in taking away our business. They were lifesavers.

All Scott's bills were sent to CCS. We went to its offices once a year with our income tax returns and any of Scott's bills that had not gone directly to them. The bills would be added up, the total subtracted from our income, and if the result was less than its tables of what a family of four needed to live on, the CCS would continue to pay Scott's bills. One year when Scott had no treatments for several months, we were put on a pay-back plan and we paid $46 a month for a year and a half. Scott's medical and hospital bills would have come to something like $50,000 if we had had to pay them ourselves.

So financially, thanks to CCS, we were all right. Physically and emotionally, I was a wreck. And Ronnie and Steven suffered considerable emotional strain. After Dr.

Martin told us that Scott had Hodgkin's, I started waking up at three or four in the morning. I would rush to the bathroom and spend half an hour vomiting and crying. Then, weak and sweating, I would slip back into bed trying not to wake Ronnie and lie rigidly awake until daylight.

Food seemed to stick in my throat and all I could think about was how Scott had complained that it hurt to swallow. I felt terribly guilty that I had not remembered that difficulty in swallowing was one of the seven warning signals of cancer. But Scott had complained about this for weeks, and nothing had clicked in my head. I kept thinking that if only I had remembered this was a warning signal, we might have caught the disease before it reached Stage Four.

The vomiting got worse when I was in Los Angeles, and one morning when Ronnie was there, I woke early as usual and rushed to the bathroom. When I came out, Ronnie was sitting up in bed.

"This goes on every morning?" he asked. I nodded. "Well, you can't go on this way. You have to eat and you have to keep food down. If you don't, you're going to get really sick and that won't help Scott. If you don't get better, you'll have to come home."

I started crying. "Please don't make me go home. I'll start eating. I promise."

When Ronnie got back to Fillmore, he called our doctor who prescribed a mild tranquilizer, and the next night Ronnie drove back to Los Angeles with the filled prescription. I had never taken a tranquilizer and could not believe that a tiny pill could restore my appetite and calm my stomach. But it helped. I started to eat more and vomit less, although the nausea never completely disappeared. All that really mattered to me was that I was well enough to be with Scott. He needed me.

In many ways these weeks were the hardest on Ronnie.

I had him to lean upon, but Ronnie had no one. When he came to Los Angeles, he always appeared strong and calm and confident. It was not until later that he told me that he was in a state of shock most of the time.

It was hard on Steven, too. He stayed with his grandparents and occasionally with friends. He did not even see Ronnie very much, because between work and his trips to Los Angeles, his dad had very little time for him. Scott and I used to talk to him on the telephone every night, but that was a poor substitute for having your mother and brother at home.

It had not been an easy time for any of us. But now we were home again. And just that fact made life sweet. We exchanged smiles and hugs and kisses more warmly than we ever had. And when Scott told us a few days after coming home that "It doesn't hurt so much to swallow," we felt a surge of happiness. It was the first good sign. We were sure there would be many more, but then one morning he called me into his room. "Mom, there's a lump at the top of my incision," he said, full of fear. I could feel the lump. And I was sure I knew what it meant. The cancer was spreading.

"Let's have Dad take a look," I said. Ronnie came in and felt the lump. "Oh, that's just scar tissue," he said, and relief spread over Scott's face like the sun coming up. Later I asked Ronnie if he was sure that it was just scar tissue. "No," he said, "but I don't want Scott to be scared. It's important that we give him an answer right away that will reassure him. I don't want him to be afraid—even when I am."

I made notes on everything, so when we saw Dr. Williams at the outpatient clinic on December 27, I could report accurately on Scott's progress. I wrote down how Scott saw yellow dots in front of his eyes. And how on December 19, his hair started to fall out. And how, two days before Christmas, Scott told me that "swallowing hurts as bad as it did in the beginning." I could hardly wait for the appointment with Dr. Williams.

I packed the car the night before we went to Childrens, something that was to become routine through the years —a pillow and blanket so Scott could lie down in the back on the way home, a thermos of water, a pan in case he threw up. Scott took paper and pencils and an armful of books. He loved to read, and books became his defense against the noise and frustrations of the clinic. When he was absorbed in a book, he was oblivious to the rest of the world. Steven was the same way. Once when Steven went to the clinic with us, a new hematologist was to examine Scott. He asked us to wait a few minutes so he could go through Scott's file and "see just where he is in terms of treatment." The two boys started reading. After a few minutes, the doctor said, "I'm sorry to keep you waiting, but I needed to go way back and . . ." He stopped and gave a kind of startled look at Steven and Scott, who had not glanced up. "Do they always read that intensely?" he asked. I nodded. "They're really something," he said to me when he finally put the chart down, ready to start the examination.

The first part of our drive to Los Angeles was along a country road with walnut and avocado groves on one side and the Santa Clara River on the other. Scott always tried to see how many birds and animals he could identify along this stretch. There were three hawks at one bend in the river that got to be old friends. Sometimes Scott would ask me to stop for a few minutes so he could walk along the river. When we hit the freeway, Scott would reach for a book or his writing pad and stay busy until we reached the hospital.

Once at Childrens, it was wait, wait, wait. That first day we stood in line for half an hour after we arrived at eight. When we were second in line, the clerk who was collecting the appointment slips closed the window and put up a sign that it would open again at 8:45. It was almost nine before I handed her Scott's appointment slip. She glanced at it, filled out a few other forms, and without even looking at me, thrust them through the window, saying, "Take these to the clerk around the corner." The next clerk took a pink form from the bunch and, again without looking at me, instructed me to put it in a box on the wall. We waited in the corridor until Scott's name was called. Another unsmiling woman drew blood from his arm and directed him to go across the hall and get weighed and measured.

Then we spotted a room down the hall where children were sitting at tables, coloring and playing games. Scott settled down with a group of children who were cutting and pasting. Suddenly I heard my name. A woman introduced herself and said she'd like to talk with me. I explained that I was waiting for Scott's appointment with Dr. Williams.

"Oh, that's all right. I'll leave word at the desk that you are with me. Someone will come for you when the doctor is ready. You don't mind leaving Scott here, do you?"

"Oh, no," I said, "my aunt is with us."

"I'm sorry I didn't talk with you when Scott was hospitalized," she said, "but I was on vacation." There was a big box of tissues on the corner of her desk nearest me. I decided she must be a psychologist.

"Does it bother you to drive here alone?" she asked abruptly.

I shook my head. "Why?"

"I wondered, since your aunt is with you."

I explained that I had asked my Aunt Hazel to come with us this first day because I didn't know what to expect at the clinic and didn't want to leave Scott alone in case Dr. Williams wanted to talk with me. "I didn't know that there was a playroom and a volunteer in charge," I told her.

"How are you and your husband," she referred to the file in front of her, "—uh, Ronnie, handling your problem?"

I told her that we were managing and that we were optimistic about Scott's recovery.

"You understand that Scott has Stage Four Hodgkin's disease, don't you?"

"Yes."

"You understand what that means, don't you?" she asked abruptly.

"Yes," I answered again. Of course I understood what it meant. It was why I woke up feeling nauseous every morning, why I cried myself to sleep every night. Ronnie and I checked each of the boys before we went to bed. We would watch Scott sleeping, so innocent, trusting that he was going to be cured. We would think of what Stage Four meant and try not to believe what the doctors had told us. It was killing me a little every day. I did not tell her this. But, yes, I knew what Stage Four Hodgkin's meant.

After a few more questions, she said, "Please call me if you have any problems I can help you with." I could not imagine anything that she could help me with. Somehow I felt inadequate around her, maybe because I thought that she disapproved of the way I was handling things.

Finally it was time for Scott to see Dr. Williams. It was like seeing an old friend. He checked Scott's nodes, listened to his lungs and heart, took his blood pressure, looked into his eyes, tested his reflexes, and asked him how he was and how it felt to be home. And he told me that there was nothing to worry about—not the yellow dots, not the lump at the top of the incision, not the renewed difficulty in swallowing.

"We'll start the second course of treatment today," he

said. "I'll make an appointment for you to come back
next week for the second injection." In the treatment
room, we found another old friend, Dr. Barak, the hematologist. He asked Scott how he'd been feeling and what
he'd got for Christmas and gave him the choice of having
his treatment, sitting up or lying down. Dr. Williams and
Dr. Barak were a welcome contrast to all the unsmiling
clerks and technicians who had treated us like objects
instead of people all morning. For weeks their imper-
sonal brusqueness alternately hurt and infuriated me,
until I decided that it was simply their defense against
the heartbreak of seeing gravely ill children and their
mothers day after day after day. They could not let themselves get involved.

These clinic visits were to form the counterpoint to
our daily life for the next four years. The time of day
varied, the intervals between visits varied, but the routine was always the same. And when we were back in the
car heading toward the freeway, heading toward home,
we always felt a sense of deliverance even though Scott
would probably start vomiting on the way home and be
sick for the next few days.

Now that he was home, Scott fought taking his pills
even more than he had in the hospital. Ronnie and I
decided that it was a good sign, that he felt stronger.
Nevertheless I dreaded pill time. There were days when
he would take them without a fuss, but others when he'd
not be able to swallow them unless he had a certain drink
to wash them down with a certain cookie to kill the taste.
Only milk and crackers would do. Or was it apple juice
and Oreos? Or orange juice and Mallomars? Whatever it
was, nothing else would do.

One night at a restaurant, I put Scott's pills beside his
plate. He ignored them. When it was time to order dessert, I told him he had to take his pills first. He started

arguing that they tasted so awful he couldn't get them down until he had his dessert.

"They can't be all that bad," Ronnie said. "Just pop them in your mouth and wash them down with the rest of your milk."

"They're horrible, Dad! They're just awful!"

"Worse than aspirin?"

"A thousand times worse," Scott stated solemnly.

"I don't believe it," Ronnie told him. "Here, give me one." Scott picked a white pill off the paper napkin where I had put his four suppertime pills and Ronnie chewed up the pill.

"That's not so bad," he said. "No worse than aspirin. And I didn't even have anything to wash it down with. What's the big deal? You don't even have to chew them. I don't see what's so horrible and awful."

Scott was impressed. The remaining three pills went down without further protest. As we walked out to the car afterward, I asked Ronnie, "How did it really taste?"

"A thousand times worse than aspirin," he answered sheepishly.

There were times when I would have to stand by Scott's bed at night and make sure that he got the last of his daily twelve pills down. "You don't have to stand there and stare at me," he would grumble. He was always the most difficult after his treatments. One day he was so angry when I insisted he take his pills that he kicked a door—and bruised his foot. The next time we went to the clinic, Dr. Williams spotted the bruise. "How did you get that black-and-blue mark, Scott?"

"Oh, I kicked a door," Scott said, giving me a smile.

"You had a little temper tantrum, huh?" Dr. Williams commented. Later he told me that depression and mood swings were side effects of the drugs.

The treatments were doing Scott good. His appetite

had improved and he had gained a few pounds. Each time we went to the clinic, Dr. Williams would say, "Well, Scott's blood count is staying up. We can keep on with the treatment."

There were a lot of questions that I wanted to ask him. I wanted to know if the fact that the blood count was staying up meant that now Scott might have more than two years to live. I wanted to know just how he thought Scott was doing. But he was always so busy that I hesitated to ask. I would think—well, he'll tell me if it's anything I should know.

We had been at the clinic three or four times and I still had not heard the results of Scott's liver biopsy. One day when Dr. Williams handed me Scott's prescriptions and started to walk away, I decided that I just had to ask him. I raced down the hall after him.

"Dr. Williams?" He turned. "Did you get the results of the liver biopsy?"

"Oh, yes. It was positive," he said quickly.

"Positive?"

"Yes." And he turned and walked off.

I felt as if the breath had been knocked out of me. I fought for control. Dear God, don't let me start crying. I felt indignant, too. I should not have been given this news in a crowded hall. He should have told me in private. It would have hurt just as much, but I would not have had to fight so hard to stay calm in front of Scott. I was sure this was what Dr. Williams had asked Dr. Gates to tell me that last day Scott had been in the hospital. He must have thought I had known all this time. I was just not ready for his answer. As I had not been ready for so many of the truths that I had been given about Scott's illness.

Scott had his own questions and he was not hesitant about asking them. One day he asked Dr. Williams, "If I have Hodgkin's, why am I coming to the Hematology Clinic?"

Dr. Williams glanced at me. Then he answered, "We've found that the drugs used to treat leukemia and other blood diseases are effective with Hodgkin's, too."

Chapter Four

THE mothers who filled the waiting room of the Hematology-Oncology Clinic at Childrens came there week after week, month after month—some of them, like me, year after year. We watched our children's hair fall out from the treatments, watched them grow thinner and paler, watched their cheeks swell chipmunk-plump from the drugs, watched a blessed few grow strong and rosy. A mother and child would disappear for a few weeks, then come back, and the child would be shockingly changed, weaker, whiter, closer to death. One day we would realize that we had not seen them for a long while. And knew we would never see them again.

Most of us went through the same experiences, were beset by the same fears and loneliness. Most of us felt uncomfortable in the hospital. We were too timid to ask the busy doctors and nurses what we wanted to know. We shared the same desperation when our children were in pain. And most of us had personal problems in addition to our sick child who absorbed our strength, our thoughts, our emotions almost completely. As the years went by, I became aware of divorces, separations, runaway children, attempted suicides. Catastrophic, long-term illness destroys more than the principal victim.

Scott and I shared the world of the clinic waiting room. It was as real to us as our own living room. It made for a schizophrenic kind of life. When we left Fillmore for Los Angeles, we moved into another world that Ronnie and Steven did not share with us. Could not, even though both occasionally accompanied us. We described it to them. They listened sensitively. But it was a world that did not take on reality until you were in it. It was as if Scott and I entered one of those old-fashioned paper-weight scenes where we could see out and others could see in, but they could not enter—and we could never completely emerge. Even at home, the shadow of the waiting room was behind us or ahead of us.

I was glad that Ronnie and Steven were not part of it. Ronnie was the anchor in my life. If he had been as involved in the immediacy of the treatment and the clinic world, he would not have been able to have been as strong for me as he was. And Steven—dear, good, cheerful Steven—was Scott's anchor. He kept him in touch with childhood, with school, and with their friends. He kept him from being a victim of my sometimes exaggerated worries.

The other mothers in the waiting room community proved to be islands of comfort and stability. A few days after Scott's staging operation, a boy moved in to share his room—and I made a new friend. Richard had been in Childrens before. His leukemia had been diagnosed a year ago. Now he was back on Four West for transfusions and medicine to fight an infection. His mother Joanne became a great source of comfort to me. We discovered that we had reacted the same way to many of our hospital experiences. She also had been unable to eat after the doctors told her that Richard had leukemia. She also had kept hoping against hope that the tests were faulty. It meant so much for me to talk with someone who knew what I was going through, what Scott was going through. To talk with another mother.

I told Joanne how scared I had been one night when I

was walking back to the motel from the hospital close to midnight and a car had drawn up beside me and stopped. All the stories I had ever heard about what can happen to lone women on deserted city streets flashed through my mind and I ran the rest of the way to the motel—a fifty-yard dash. After that I drove to the hospital parking lot every morning and back to the motel at night.

And Joanne told me how she and her husband had eaten in a restaurant across the street from the hospital for weeks because no one had told them that they could eat in the hospital cafeteria.

These incidents may seem trivial, but when everything is strange and you are worried out of your mind about your child, things like this are almost more than you can cope with. It was good to have someone to talk with and learn that I was not the only one who found this hospital world uncomfortable and bewildering. We agreed that it was not much use to ask the nurses questions. Both of us had been intimidated by tart replies to our first questions. We also realized that much of their brusqueness was due to the work load. We would much rather have them caring for our children than answering our questions.

Not all the nurses were brusque. By no means. There were many wonderful women and men on Four West. I will be forever grateful to the nurse who, after Scott's lymphangiogram, asked if I would be spending the night with him.

"Can I? Is it all right?"

"Of course you can," the nurse said warmly. "Lots of parents stay after their children have had surgery. You can sleep on the couch in his room. Just ask one of the night nurses for a blanket and a pillow."

Later I saw Joanne often in the clinic, and Richard and Scott were always pleased to see each other. One day

I asked Joanne what she and her husband had told Richard about his disease. "He knows he has leukemia," she said. "We did not tell him how serious it was. But then we needed blood donors. The newspaper ran an appeal for blood saying that he was a dying boy. And Richard read it."

"Oh." I caught my breath. What that child must have felt. "What did you tell him?" I asked.

"We said that leukemia was a very serious disease. And that some people die from it. But we also told him that newspapers tend to exaggerate when they run this kind of story, because they hope to get more response that way. We told him that new treatments were being discovered all the time. And at the end, I said, 'You know, Richard, no one knows when he is going to die.' Somehow that seemed to make sense to him."

Her story gave me courage to tell her about the nurse in charge of Four West who—before the staging operation —had asked me why I had not told Scott he had Hodgkin's. I explained that I wanted to wait until all the tests were completed.

"It is much better to tell them the truth," she said.

"I'm going to tell him the truth, but I don't think this is the right time."

"Scott is preoccupied with death," the nurse said. "Anyone can see that from his drawings. You can't hide the facts from these children. They guess the truth anyway."

She was talking about the ghosts and monsters that Scott had been drawing since before Halloween. He had made the same kind of drawings in the Ventura hospital, and Steven was turning out similar ghosts and monsters at home. Every Halloween the boys spent a lot of time making scary drawings. Scott's were no more and no less frightening than the ones he had done the year before. I could understand why the nurse thought Scott was preoccupied with death, but the monster pictures did not alarm me in the least. I knew Scott was a little scared, but I was certain that he was not preoccupied with thoughts of death. I would have known. I thought I would have known.

I told Joanne about the psychologist who had asked if he could talk with Scott before the staging operation. I asked him if he thought I should tell Scott he had cancer. He said that I should, that I should tell him everything I knew about what he had. I was immediately sorry I had asked him. In a way it might have been easier to tell Scott then, before the staging operation, before Dr. Williams had told us that Scott had only two years to live. But now? How could I tell Scott everything I knew? Could that psychologist truly think it wise to tell Scott how gravely ill he was? That the doctors had told us he would die? I wondered if the psychologist had a child of his own.

Joanne and I both agreed that it would be harmful to paint a dark picture for our sons. Who has the right to tell another person he is going to die? Who has the right to rob a human being of hope?

Since Ronnie and I had decided not to tell Scott that he had cancer, we lived in fear that someone else would tell him. We had told our friends that Scott had Hodgkin's, but not that it was Stage Four. One day a friend told me that when Scott's illness was diagnosed, his Sunday-school teacher told the class, "We know what Scott has now. He has cancer." And she asked the class to pray for him. I was very upset and called the teacher. I asked her to refer to Scott's illness as Hodgkin's. She promised that she would and that she would tell the other Sunday-school teachers to do the same.

A few weeks after Scott returned to school, he came home one afternoon and said, "Mom, do you know if I'd gotten Hodgkin's a few years ago, I'd be dead by now?"

I was working at the kitchen sink. Thankful my back was turned to Scott so that he could not see the panic in my face, I said, "No, where did you hear that?"

"I read it in the encyclopedia at school. The encyclopedia said Hodgkin's is always fatal, but the copyright date was a couple of years old."

I told him what the doctors had told us—that chemotherapy advances had been so rapid that, by the time anything about Hodgkin's was printed, it was already out of date—and that Dr. Williams had told us that there was practically nothing written about childhood Hodgkin's since it was so very rare.

"I guess I'm lucky," Scott said.

Since so many people at Childrens disagreed with me about not telling Scott he had cancer, I called Dr. Martin in Ventura and asked what he thought. "I don't think it's necessary to tell him," he said. Then I asked Dr. Williams when I should tell Scott that Hodgkin's was cancer.

"When he asks," Dr. Williams said. I wished I had asked him sooner. His matter-of-fact answer was the kind of reassurance I needed.

No mother in the waiting room community would ever have insisted or even advised that another mother tell her child he or she had cancer. This little world had its own unwritten laws. You would never ask, "Does your child have leukemia?" Instead, your first question would be something like, "How long have you been coming to Childrens?" And then, "Who's your doctor?"

We all became experts. I could soon tell what kind of cancer a child had just by the drugs he or she was taking. We talked about Wilms's tumor and Ewing's tumor and histiocytosis and neuroblastoma the way other women talk about specials at the supermarket. Somehow just being able to talk about cancer made it seem a little less frightening and more manageable.

One woman told me it helped her to see the other children. "When I first came here," she said, "I used to look at each child and think— Is that going to happen to my Cheryl? Today, I can still hope because I have seen so many children who look worse."

I thought to myself that her child must look pretty good—and then Cheryl came over to show her mother a picture she had colored. Cheryl was one of the children I had looked at and wondered— Is that going to happen to my Scott? To me she was a pathetic-looking child. But not to her mother. I discovered that most of the time we saw our children as they looked before illness struck, not as they really looked.

There were few mothers who accepted that their child would die. Joanne was one of the few. She knew Richard was going to die and she accepted it. She was always calm. I thought that somehow her acceptance gave her a reservoir of strength. I never saw her upset the way most of us were from time to time.

There were days when I would sit in the clinic waiting for Scott to have his tests and not be able to talk to anyone. I did not want to hear about low blood counts or children throwing up blood or going blind. I would hold my book in front of me and not look up, even though the print was swimming in front of my eyes. But most of the time, I looked forward to talking with the others. This was such a terrible and frightening experience and all of us women were going through it together. We were the only ones who knew what it was really like.

This may have been why there were so many family breakups and divorces. My friend Joanne's husband left her just before Richard died. They had two other wonderful, healthy children, but her husband had left. And

Joanne had to cope with a fatherless home, a dying child, and her own emotions. She was very reserved and said little about her problems, but seeing her grow thinner and more strained week after week was enough to make one realize the burdens she was carrying.

Another woman I knew also got divorced. Her whole being was centered on her daughter who had acute lymphoblastic leukemia, just as my attention was centered on Scott. One day she burst into tears and told me her husband was seeing another woman. "But I can't blame him," she said. "It's all my fault."

She told me that she had completely lost interest in sex. "I never feel like it anymore," she said. "But he hasn't tried lately, and last night he told me he wants a divorce."

There was nothing to say. No comfort to give. All I could do was listen and hope that it helped her to have someone to talk to. I could understand. All those weeks that Scott was in the hospital, sex was unthinkable for me. I was so exhausted and frantic with worry that I had no energy. Once Scott came home, things eased up and our life came back to normal. But there were to be times in the future when I thought of this woman.

Katy, whose daughter had leukemia, was having similar problems. Sex had become very rare in her marriage. "I used to be very eager," she told me, "but now—" and she shrugged her shoulders. She started going to a psychiatrist to see if he could help her and it turned into a very unpleasant episode. He told her that her marital problems stemmed from the fact that she was sexually unresponsive —just what she had told him. He assured her that he could cure this. I am sure that this psychiatrist did not know that almost all the mothers in the Hematology-Oncology Clinic suffered from sexual unresponsiveness from time to time in varying degrees. And that the cure would have been to see our children cured. The psychiatrist told Katy to read erotic books and make up sex fantasies. At each session, he would ask her to talk about her fantasies and each time he would become more sexually aggressive, going from a kiss on the cheek to a close embrace in a matter of weeks. At that point, she stopped going to him.

It helped us to talk. These experiences alerted me to possible dangers ahead. I could see that this could easily happen to Ronnie and me, something that would have seemed impossible a year ago. But now everything was changed. Our whole life was different. I resolved that I would not run the danger of sacrificing my marriage, no matter how terrified I was about Scott. We were to have our ups and downs during the years that Scott was sick, but I think these object lessons helped me keep my perspective. Ronnie and my marriage were too precious to be sacrificed to cancer.

Not every woman at the clinic was friendly or compatible or even likable. Some were so ravaged by their child's illness that they hated the world and everyone in it. But most of the members of the waiting room community, a fluid community whose population shifted from month to month, were strong women, staunch women who looked death in the eye and dared it to take their child. In a way we became each other's second family, a family bonded by illness and death, a family that existed only within the confines of the clinic, but a family nevertheless.

Chapter Five

THERE was a delicious feeling of everything getting
back to normal. I had never realized just how happy we
had been before Scott's illness, how good the comfortable
humdrum of our life had been. Not until everything was
shaken up and we were all just hanging on for dear life
hoping to struggle through. And it began to look as if perhaps we had struggled through.

Scott went back to school after Christmas. His fifth-
grade teacher, Mrs. Padelford, had sacrificed a good part
of her Christmas vacation tutoring Scott so he would be
able to keep up with the others. Both boys had belonged
to the school band. Scott played the trumpet, Steven the
drums, and Scott wanted to get back in the band. But he
did not have the lung power to play the trumpet anymore. The band teacher suggested that he play the
drums, although there were already more drummers in
the band than he needed. Steven taught Scott what he
knew until he caught up with the other drummers. Sometimes it got pretty noisy at 644 Saratoga Street, but I
loved the racket. It meant both boys were happy and
busy—and together. When I used to see Scott hauling that
big drum to school, I had to smile. It was almost as big as
he was. The first band concert Steven and Scott played in

was very special for us. Watching them thumping away at the drums made Ronnie and me feel that everything was going to be all right no matter what the doctors said.

Steven's helping Scott learn to play the drum was just one of many ways he helped his brother. He was very concerned about Scott, even though there were times when he felt left out of things because Scott absorbed so much of our attention. But I made a point now of taking time to have long talks with Steven. I told him over and over that we had hated to leave him alone so much while Scott was in the hospital, but that there hadn't been anything else for us to do. I told him that if he ever felt hurt and out of things because it seemed as if we were paying more attention to Scott, he should tell me. I told him that his dad and I loved him very much and we appreciated the way he had adapted himself to the situation and helped make things easier for us. These were things he needed to hear more than once. Scott *was* getting more attention. And it was too much to expect ten-year-old Steven to take this all in his stride. But as the weeks went by and Scott got stronger, our lives slowly returned to their former course and there was very little difference between Scott and Steven.

They were old enough to join the Boy Scouts, but I worried that Scott would not be well enough to keep up with the others on their hikes and camping trips, especially after he had been in Los Angeles for his treatments. The scoutmaster reassured me, saying, "Scott can participate just as much as he feels he can. There won't be any problems." But I still worried.

The first overnight hike found me in a tizzy. Ronnie tried to calm me. "They'll be fine," he said. "If anything's wrong, they'll bring Scott home. They're not all that far away." But I kept worrying. Scott might be cold. He might not feel well. He might want to come home and hesitate to say so. That night I talked Ronnie into driving me to the campsite. I rushed over to the Scout leader and asked how Scott was. "Quit worrying about him," he told me. "He's fine. He's out getting firewood with Steven and some other kids." And Ronnie said, "Come on. Let's get out of here before he gets back and sees us." I felt very foolish on the way home, but I didn't care. I just had to be sure that Scott was all right.

I probably should have worried more about Steven at that time. I was to discover that he had a lot of fears that he never mentioned. When Scott was too weak from his treatment or had a cold and could not make one of the Scout overnight hikes, Steven got sick too. He would go off with the other boys, but every morning he would be sick to his stomach. When I asked him about it, he would say, "Oh, Mom, I just ate too many pancakes for breakfast," or, "I took too many salt pills," but this only happened when Steven went off alone. At the time I did not feel that I should poke and pry at Steven, so I decided to say nothing unless there were other developments. In a way, I thought I understood it. The boys had always done everything together, and although they sometimes fought with each other, they were very close. Steven had become terribly considerate and careful of Scott since his illness. He worried about him a lot. And that was enough to make a person sick, as I knew from my own experience.

Steven used to wake up in the middle of the night and go into Scott's room to see if he was all right. Scott's room was in the front of the house, Steven's in the middle, and ours at the back. Steven was afraid that if Scott needed something, we could not hear him call out.

"I'd go in Scott's room," Steven told one of his friends, "and he'd be tossing around in bed. Sometimes he'd be saying something in his sleep and then he'd wake up with a yell or a groan." But when Scott woke up and found Steven there, he would be furious.

"Mom, every time I move in bed," he told me, "that

Steven runs in and wakes me up and asks if I'm all right. Tell him to quit it."

So I had a talk with Steven. I explained that Scott was stronger now and that it wasn't like when he was in the hospital and had to bang on the side of his bed when he wanted the nurse to come because he was too weak to call her. "Now he can call out," I said, "and pretty loudly, too. He could probably wake the whole neighborhood." This helped Steven relax a little.

When Scott got stronger, there was another problem. The boys had fought hard all their lives. Now they started squabbling about all the usual things. They would yell at each other and ten minutes later be the best of friends. It had always been this way. I remember once when they were little Scott was running through the house, crying. Steven was running after him, hitting him and laughing. Ronnie set out after the boys to make Steven stop, but by the time he had caught up with them, Scott was running after Steven and it was Steven who was doing the crying. Minutes later they were playing together in the backyard.

But now Steven complained that Scott would push him or hit him and he didn't dare hit back because he was afraid he'd hurt Scott.

"I don't want you hitting each other any way," I said and left it at that. But later that week when I took Steven to Ventura for a routine physical, I told Dr. Martin that Steven worried a lot about Scott. After the checkup, the doctor asked Steven if he had any questions about Scott.

"When Scott and I fight and get really mad," Steven said a little embarrassed but very earnest, "he hits me and I want to hit him back. But what I worry about is—if I hit him, could I kill him?"

I was appalled. I didn't realize that Steven had thought he might kill his brother.

"Scott is getting stronger," Dr. Martin said. "If you feel you really have to hit him back, you won't kill him. You don't have to worry about that. But you should be careful about where you hit him. His incisions are still tender."

"Oh, I'd be careful," Steven said, obviously relieved. "I know I'm stronger than he is. I just wanted to know if I could hit him in the arm when he hits me."

"I think that would be okay," Dr. Martin said seriously.

I was so pleased with the way Dr. Martin handled this that I mentioned the way Steven had been checking on Scott in the middle of the night.

"I'm afraid when I hear him cough that he might choke or something and die," Steven said.

Dr. Martin hesitated. I knew he was looking for a way to make Steven feel better. And Steven was sitting on the edge of his chair waiting for the answer. Finally the doctor said, "I can't say when anybody is going to die. You or Scott could get hit by a car when you're riding your bikes. Accidents can happen to anyone—anytime. But I can tell you one thing. You don't have to worry about Scott suddenly dying in the middle of the night. He's doing very well. You don't have to worry about him."

That night I had a talk with both boys and told Scott what Dr. Martin had said. "There are going to be new fight rules around this house," I said. "Steven says you hit him in the stomach, Scott, because you know he won't hit you back. That's not fighting fair. From now on, the rule is that if you hit Steven, he can hit you back in the same spot. So you better think twice about where you hit him. Okay?"

We tried to maintain normal relations between the boys, but it was hard. I didn't want Steven to feel guilty when he got mad at Scott. And I encouraged him to tell me when he got mad at Scott or thought we were treating him unfairly. He seldom complained. He simply became quieter and quieter. I didn't know what to do about this. I did not want to spoil Scott because he was sick, nor did I want to overreact and spoil Steven because I felt he was being neglected. Dr. Williams had told me that psychologists had found that the brothers and sisters of very ill children or of children who died often had serious psychological problems. A lot of them ran away from home.

Ronnie used to tell me that I let Scott get away with murder. And I did have a hard time cracking down on him when he misbehaved, because I knew how much pain he had been in. "I try to be fair," I told Dr. Williams, "but—well, I just find it hard to be tough with Scott."

"It's hard, I know," Dr. Williams said, "but you've got to think of Steven and be fair to him." And I tried.

I also worried that Steven might be worried that he would come down with Hodgkin's, too, even though we had told him it was unlikely. Ronnie and I had worried about this ever since Scott's illness was diagnosed. After all, they were identical twins and they had always had coughs and sniffles at the same time. One of the hematologists had told me that the chances of Steven's having Hodgkin's were about one in a hundred, but that was too big a chance for me. I still worried.

One day when Ronnie had brought Steven down to visit Scott at Childrens, Dr. Williams asked if Steven would be staying long enough so he could have some blood tests run and get a chest X ray.

"Why do you want to do those tests on me?" Steven asked a little uncertainly.

"Well, the chest X ray is just a precaution, but we'd like to see if your blood matches Scott's. If it does, we may be able to use it someday to help in Scott's treatment."

"Oh, okay," Steven agreed. He had his tests in the

morning and Dr. Gates told us she'd let us know the results as soon as possible. Hours went by. I knew that the blood tests did not take long and neither did the chest X ray. The more time that passed, the more worried I got. Finally late in the afternoon when I could not stand the uncertainty any longer, I went looking for Dr. Gates and asked when she thought she'd have the results.

"Oh," she sighed, "didn't I tell you? Steven's tests were all normal. I'm so sorry I didn't tell you earlier. I had the results this morning."

It was one of those situations where I was so relieved at the news that I did not blame Dr. Gates for neglecting to give us the report. Instead I blamed myself for not taking the initiative and asking her sooner.

When I told Steven that his tests showed that he was in good shape and had no signs of Hodgkin's, I could see he was relieved although he said nothing. I was grateful that Dr. Williams had suggested these tests.

Just when we began to feel relaxed and dare to hope that the doctors had been unduly pessimistic about Scott's chances, we had an unexpected family tragedy, one that Steven may have taken harder than anyone else.

Both boys were very close to their Grandpa Jack, Ronnie's father. His hobby was trapshooting and the boys loved it when he took them out to the dried-up riverbed to shoot their BB guns. Sometimes he'd let them use his precious .22. The boys would sit for hours listening to their grandpa talk about hunting and shooting and the great out-of-doors, things that their own dad was not the least interested in. Ronnie much preferred tinkering with his old cars—he has restored several antique cars, real showpieces—than fooling around with guns. Steven was perhaps a little closer to his Grandpa Jack because he had spent so much time with him when Scott was in the hospital.

One April evening just after the boys had gone to bed, the phone rang. It was Ronnie's mother, Roma. "Jack's awfully sick," she said. Jack was rushed to the emergency room at the hospital, but they could not save him. He had suffered a massive heart attack. He was only fifty-six and a recent checkup had shown him to be in good shape.

When we told the boys, Scott started crying, but Steven just got up and went into his room. He didn't say much and he didn't cry. Not once. But for the next two months, he was tormented by nightmares. Then one night he called me into his room. "I can't stand to think of Grandpa Jack dead. I miss him so much," he said, his voice cracking. And then the tears came. I held him the way I used to when he was little and just let him cry. It had to come out. And after that he had fewer nightmares, but he dreamed a lot about his grandpa.

They were happy dreams most of them. "I had a dream that my grandpa and I were riding around in his pickup truck," he told a friend. "I liked just riding around with him. It was like he had a reprieve from death and he was going to die again. He didn't know that he was just here for a month or two, but I did. It didn't matter. We were driving around having a good time. I was really pleased he was here.

"I dreamed this a lot. Sometimes in color, sometimes in black and white. The old truck was a '64, sort of a nondescript gray white. He wore these old beat-up pants and his heavy boots. His shotguns were in a case in the back, seven or eight guns. The best was a Winchester, a twenty-two that was made in 1916. It shoots the straightest. My dad gave it to Scott after Grandpa died and then when Scott died, I got it. But in my dream, we'd be driving down Central on our way out to the shooting range. That was all there was to it.

"It was a real short dream. I'd be sitting there in the

truck beside him being happy. And then the dream would be over."

Somehow we managed to get over Jack's death. Roma came back to work in the store. Keeping busy helped her, and Ronnie kept himself extra busy, too. I started working more hours to help out. And Scott would drop by after school for an hour or so. Ronnie taught him how to run the cash register and he used to ring up sales and make change.

Scott was really getting better. That spring he and Steven went hiking in the hills. Sometimes they brought home fossils they had discovered. Once they came back with dozens of polliwogs that they watched turn into frogs and then let loose in Sespe Creek, not far from our house on the edge of the Los Padres National Forest. The rest of the school year was like moving in and out of the sunshine. Scott was doing well in school and having fun, then he would have to go to the clinic for his injection. That was like moving into the shadow. He would start worrying about it a couple of days before, then there would be the long day at the clinic and the long drive home. The drive home was longer because the nausea often attacked him and we would have to stop while he vomited, but as he got stronger, the vomiting after his treatments became less severe and then disappeared. On balance, there seemed to be more sunshine than shadow in our lives.

All this time I had been praying for Scott to be cured. Then I read about miracles that had taken place after people had totally and sincerely submitted their problems to God's will, saying that they would accept whatever God did because it was His will. So after much struggling with my belief in God and with my love for Scott and my desire that he be cured, I stopped asking God to make him well. I decided that if I really believed in God, then I had to tell Him I was willing for Him to take Scott if that was His will. And I did. There were tears in my eyes as I prayed, but I had to believe that God was love.

And the miracle took place. On our next clinic visit, Dr. Williams smiled and said, "Well, good news. Scott's X rays are the best ever this time." God had heard me. God's will was being done. God was love.

"Can I stop the treatments?" Scott wanted to know.

"No, we want to give you a few more," Dr. Williams said. I was sure that after a few more treatments Scott would be well. I had good reason to believe this.

Our neighbors, Jeff and Lulu Page, had met a couple named Russell when they were camping out the previous summer and learned that their son Duane had Hodgkin's. The Russells told Lulu that everyone had thought Duane would die, but that he was fine. Lulu wrote to them about Scott after the doctors told us he had Hodgkin's, and Gladys Russell wrote me a warm, encouraging letter telling about Duane.

The doctors at Stanford Medical Center had diagnosed his Hodgkin's at Stage Four—just like Scott's—and the Russells had been told that Duane had only a short time to live. He had a lymph node in his neck the size of an orange. But Duane had been healed. By God. He was one of the first patients at Stanford to be given chemotherapy, but even before the treatments started, that lymph node had begun to shrink.

The Russells had prayed for their son and so had many other people. Mr. Russell wrote about Duane's cure in *The Pentecostal Evangel.* "Our niece phoned," he wrote, "to give us two Scripture verses which the believers felt the Lord had given them especially for us—

'I have heard thy prayer, I have seen thy tears: Behold, I will heal thee.' —Kings 2, 20:5

'Let not your heart be troubled,
Neither let it be afraid.' —John 14:27

"We eagerly grasped these promises," Mr. Russell
wrote, "and that night the Lord gave us great peace and
calmness. The next morning we awakened, knowing that
somehow Duane would be healed."

Even though the Russells knew that God was healing
Duane and would cure him, they felt the Lord wanted
Duane to receive the chemotherapy treatments and so
they signed the consent forms. His disease had been diagnosed in December 1969, almost two years before Scott's.
He had received chemotherapy for six months, and all his
symptoms had disappeared before the end of the treatment.

Duane is married now and still free of Hodgkin's. He
goes to the Stanford Medical Center once a year for a
checkup. The doctors there call him their "miracle boy."

I told Dr. Williams about Duane. He wanted to know
if he had been given radiotherapy as well as chemotherapy. "No," I told him, "the doctors felt his disease
was too widespread for radiation. He got the same drugs
that Scott is taking." Dr. Williams just nodded. I wondered what he thought about the case. Later that day, I
overheard him talking to another doctor. I caught just a
few words ". . . and she said the boy didn't have any
radiation, just chemotherapy." I was tempted to inter-
rupt and tell him that I was certain now that Scott was
going to make it, but I didn't quite dare.

We had a lot of telephone calls from people who
wanted us to take Scott to healers. And a surprising number of people came to the house urging us to take Scott
off all treatment. One woman whose son was being
treated for leukemia in Mexico gave me directions on
how to get to the Mexican clinic and strongly suggested

that I take Scott there as soon as possible. Another woman told me to take him to Kathryn Kuhlman, the healer. I resisted all these suggestions. At least three quarters of the mothers at the clinic had tried some form of spiritual healing for their children, and a few children— something like five percent—had gone into spontaneous remission. But Dr. Williams told me that they could count on that same percentage of spontaneous remissions without faith healing. I felt that God heard my prayers and those of our family and friends. (I had been amazed at how many people would come into the store—people who were not churchgoers—and say, "I'm praying for you." It made me change some of my ideas. I realized that your relationship with God does not depend on how much you go to church.) I had faith in God and did not feel that I had to seek Him through a particular person. And Scott himself had faith.

When Scott and Steven were baptized, they had to stand up and give their reasons for wanting to live as Christians. Scott said, "I want to be a Christian and live as God would want me to, since He's been so good to me."

One day when Scott was lying on the living room couch after his treatment, he said, "Mom, I know why God has let me have Hodgkin's disease. It was so I would learn compassion, understanding, and consideration of others."

I didn't know what to say. Could he possibly have been right?

By the end of the fifth grade, Scott had improved so much that it was just about unbelievable. He had gone on overnight hikes with the Scouts. He had done well in school, even though he had to miss a few days every month because of his treatments. The last day of school, he gave his teacher a little gift with a card he had made.

He had drawn a skinny little mouse on the front of the card; when you opened it up, there was a fat mouse nibbling on a piece of cheese. "I decided the skinny mouse was how Scott thought of himself when he came back to school," his teacher told me, "and the bouncy, fat mouse the way he felt at the end of school."

Then began what was perhaps the best summer of our lives. Every day seemed golden. The boys and their friends were in and out of the swimming pool all day. We went on short hikes up Sespe Creek. We spent a couple of weeks at the beach with Ronnie's mother. We had friends over for cookouts at the pool. We were all relaxed in a way that had not been possible during the long, frightening winter. Except for clinic days, it was almost possible to forget that Scott was ill. He was gaining weight and looked tan and healthy.

The highlight of the summer was a week-long camping trip late in August. Parents were invited to accompany the Scouts. Dr. Williams saw no reason why Scott should not go, so the four of us took off for Horseshoe Lake in the High Sierra for what turned out to be seven freezing cold days. I worried constantly that Scott would catch cold. At night around the campfire, I would ask Scott how he was. "I'm fine, Mom. I'm plenty warm," he'd assure me. And he seemed to be. He went along on all the hikes and outings, did his share of the work, and enjoyed himself thoroughly.

The big event of the week was a father-son overnight hike higher up in the mountains. I shivered all night in my sleeping bag and wondered how Ronnie and the boys were doing. The next day I watched the Scouts and their weary fathers straggle back. Scott was bright and chipper. He told me cheerfully that they had woken in the morning to find their sleeping bags covered with frost.

As we left Horseshoe Lake at the end of the week, snow

started to fall, something that made a big impression on the boys since we rarely saw snow in Fillmore. It was the perfect ending to a wonderful summer.

On our next visit to the clinic, several doctors came around to ask Scott about his rugged camping trip. Ronnie had been very proud of the way Scott had kept up with the others on the overnight hike, but I had thought he was just being a typical doting dad until I listened to the doctors discuss with some wonderment what Scott had been able to do. To me, this indicated that he was doing better than expected—and would be cured.

Chapter Six

Iᴛ ᴡᴀs just a year since Scott had first complained about trouble in swallowing—a heartrending, miserable year. But things were better now. The treatments were helping. And now Scott was starting sixth grade along with Steven.

All summer, Scott had pursued what he referred to as "my interests" quite diligently. His interests were varied, but his chief one was World War Two. Scott had been so caught up in reading about the war and collecting memorabilia that the first day he had been hospitalized in Ventura, Ronnie had gone looking for a special present to cheer him up—and there was no question but that it had to be something military—and had come back with a set of captain's bars. This had pleased Scott tremendously. "Now I can order the nurses not to stick me," he said with his impish, little-boy smile.

In sixth grade, Scott's interest in World War Two really took off. He and his dad spent most Sundays at swap meets where Ronnie looked for parts for the 1934 Ford he was restoring and Scott for military items. These days everyone in Fillmore knows Ronnie's 1934 Ford. It's a bright pink sedan with running boards. He drives it to the store every day. But in those days it was a pretty sorry mess. Steven once described it quite accurately as a "jockey-style car. The engine's shot. There's no front hood. It has no gas pedal, steering wheel, top, rumble or driver seats, no good pressure, no speed or gas gauges, no paint and no upholstery whatsoever. Not to mention no wheels. It's a rotted piece of junk."

Even though Scott was more interested in the car than Steven, once he got to the swap meets, he spent his time looking for military treasures and not parts for the Ford. He studied military books so he would know what items were worth buying, and he spent most of his allowance on old canteens and gun belts and hats and all kinds of military decorations and medals. At one of the first swap meets he went to, Scott found a medal he wanted, but the dealer would not sell it to him without his father's permission. So Ronnie stood by as Scott and the dealer came to an agreement on the price. Then Ronnie said, "Scott knows the value of these things better than I do. After this, whatever he agrees to is fine with me."

That fall the boys met a man who opened up a whole new world to them. Steven had become interested in taxidermy. He had read everything the library had on the subject. Now he wanted to try "stuffing" a bird. I suggested that he first consult Webb McKelvey, the proprietor of the Sespe Taxidermy Shop, so one day after school, the boys and I went to the shop. I was impressed when I saw the specimens Webb had mounted. He showed Steven the detailed sketches he made before he touched a specimen and gave him all kinds of advice on how to start. The boys were fascinated by everything in the shop and even more fascinated by Webb's stories about animals and their habitats. After this, the boys often went to his shop just to talk. Webb told them about the animals he saw hiking along Sespe into the mountains. And sometimes he came by the house in his truck

SCOTT WAS HERE 69

and took the boys into the hills to look for fossils and animal tracks.

Soon it seemed as if Scott were quoting Webb every other sentence. "You don't really have to go into the wilderness to find wildlife, you know, Mom," he would tell me. "Webb says that if a fellow just gets up early in the morning and takes a short walk along the Sespe, he can see bobcats and foxes. And in the evening, you can see quail and deer."

When Scott discovered that Webb had been badly wounded in World War Two and had spent months in the hospital and still had to return to the hospital occasionally, this solidified the bond between the two. Webb in his fifties and Scott not yet in his teens became the best of friends.

The boys were twelve in January and Ronnie and I were full of rejoicing. Scott was so well. Could this be the boy who had been given only two years to live? That had been fourteen months ago—and just look at Scott. He had gained weight, his color was good, and he had almost as much energy as Steven. If it weren't for the treatments that dragged him down every month, he would be fine.

The next time we went to the clinic, Dr. Williams ordered a complete set of X rays. "Well, Scott," he said, "we're not going to give you any injections this month." Scott sat there on the examining table and beamed. Dr. Williams said he would study the X rays, review Scott's case with the other doctors, and that we should come back in March.

When we went back to Los Angeles in March, Dr. Williams told us that one of the hematologists at Childrens was going to a conference on childhood Hodgkin's in Texas and that he wanted to wait until she got back and reported on what she had learned before making any decisions about Scott. Then he would review all the cases of childhood Hodgkin's at Childrens before he decided on Scott's future treatment. I can't describe how relieved and happy Scott was to have another month go by with no treatment. They were grim. The drugs were savage. And the injections painful. The last one in January had been particularly bad. The hematologist had looked over Scott's arm and hand, trying to find a good vein for the IV for his treatment. He made a couple of attempts, both unsuccessful. When he said he was going to have to try again, Scott groaned. Just then another hematologist walked in and asked, "What's the matter?"

"I don't want another injection."

"Why not?" she demanded.

"Because it hurts," Scott said softly.

"Well," she said cheerfully, "you're just going to have to get used to that." I think I could easily have killed her. Anyone who looked at Scott's needle-scarred arms and hands had to know that he had been "used to" injections and pain for a long time.

When we went back to the clinic in April, Dr. Williams said, "No treatment today, Scott. And no more pills." The hematologist who had gone to Texas had reported that no one had any different or better treatment for childhood Hodgkin's than Childrens, which was considered to be the largest and best treatment center for the disease. Childrens had treated twenty-five children for Hodgkin's in the past five years.

When Scott heard "no more pills," his smile lit up the room and his brown eyes shone with the purest happiness that one can imagine. That night he lit some of the sparklers he had saved from the Fourth of July for "when I'm really cured."

Now that there were no treatments hanging over him, Scott really began to enjoy life. He also began taking an interest in girls, one girl in particular. Her name was Glenda. And Glenda had a twin sister. The girls would ride their horses by our house afternoons and visit with Scott and Steven. They were inches taller than the boys, but that did not bother any of them in the slightest. Glenda and Scott exchanged charms and he wore hers on a chain around his neck.

Then one day Scott came home from school absolutely despondent. I took one look and my heart dropped. He went straight to his room, threw himself on his bed, and turned his face to the wall. I didn't know what to do. A few days before, Scott had exploded, "Quit asking me how I feel all the time! You ask me how I feel the first thing in the morning, all day long, and before I go to bed. I don't always know how I feel. And sometimes I don't want to know. When you ask me, it just makes me stop and think if I feel bad."

He was right and I promised him I would stop pestering him about it. But now I wanted to know how he felt and what was wrong. I walked past his room several times. He looked absolutely defeated. I was afraid I knew what it was— He's learned that Hodgkin's is cancer, I thought, and he's angry with me for not telling him. And he's frightened.

Finally I had to find out what was wrong. I went in and sat on his bed. "Is something wrong?"

"Yes."

"Do you want to tell me about it?"

"I just feel terrible," he said in a very depressed tone.

"Do you hurt someplace?"

"No, I'm not sick. I just feel terrible about something that happened at school."

I waited.

Then it came tumbling out. "We started this secret club. And Glenda heard about it. She wanted to join. I told her she couldn't. It's just for boys and I wasn't even supposed to talk to her about it.

"Now I'm afraid she's mad at me and won't like me anymore," he concluded miserably.

He didn't know! He still didn't know that he had cancer. I could have laughed in relief. I could have cried, too, because I still remembered what it was like to be in the sixth grade and like someone very much.

"I don't think she's really mad," I said. "And if she is a little mad, she won't stay that way. Tomorrow, why don't you tell her that you're sorry you can't talk about the club and that you hope she'll understand? I think she will."

"Really?"

"Really."

And she did.

Toward the end of the sixth grade, Scott had a run of colds and he complained that his neck and chest itched. The itching disturbed me. I had read that it was one of the symptoms of Hodgkin's. And I remembered that when he was in the third grade, there was a time when he was forever scratching his arms until they bled. I had taken him to the doctor, who had said it was probably just something he got from playing in the high grass or the bushes. Nothing to worry about.

I had asked Dr. Williams about it at one time and he had said, "It probably was some sort of allergy. We usually only see itching in adult Hodgkin's patients." When I asked him if Scott could possibly have had Hodgkin's as long ago as the third grade, he said that no one could know. "Scott could have had it for as little as two months," he said. So I put the itching out of my mind and decided not to feel guilty that I had not spotted an early symptom of Hodgkin's. But now Scott was itching again. I called Dr. Martin in Ventura and asked him about it. He said that since Scott had no other symptoms, there was no reason to suspect anything serious. "I see kids every day with the same kind of itching," he said.

During the last few weeks of school, the itching became more bothersome. And Scott complained that his neck ached. I gave him a Tylenol and that seemed to take care of it. But every afternoon, he would tell me that his neck hurt again.

In the flurry of excitement over the end of school, his symptoms seemed to disappear. His sixth-grade report was excellent and the teacher's comment made us glow with pride—"Scott has a very unique personality," she wrote. "I've learned so much from him due to all his varied interests. A very well-rounded person." On graduation day, we learned that Scott was one of the first-place winners in the American Legion Americanism Essay Contest for the second year in succession. This year he had written about the flag— "I see the colors and know what they stand for . . . The red stripes stand for bloodshed and courage, the white stripes stand for purity and truth. The blue stands for vigilance, perseverance and justice. I am proud that our country has what our flag stands for."

After school ended, we took the first family vacation we'd had since we moved back to Fillmore. We went to Catalina and had a great time going on the tours and swimming in the ocean. Scott's fun was diminished because his neck aches and backaches and the itching became more persistent. He scratched himself so much that I had to bandage his shoulders to keep him from scratching himself in his sleep.

A few days later, Scott and I were back at Childrens. I hoped Dr. Williams would know what the aches and itching were all about, but as it happened another hematologist examined Scott that day. She reported that his X rays and blood counts were good. When she left the examining room, I followed her. "I'm upset about those neck and backaches," I said. "He's in real pain at times. And that itch is driving him crazy. Do you know what's causing these?"

She shook her head. "The aches could be muscular. Or tuberculosis in his bones. I'm going to give him a TB patch test. If he still has the backaches when you come back next month, we'll do some more tests and a bone scan."

Life was full of shadows again. Those sunny days of last spring seemed far away.

Chapter Seven

EVER since Scott had started having treatments, I had been keeping a little notebook in which I jotted down the clinic appointments, the prescriptions the doctor gave us, the doses Scott was supposed to take each day, and the results of his tests. I also wrote down Scott's symptoms.

On July 28, 1973, I wrote that Scott had backaches every day, that he was usually a "little sore" in the morning, that he would ask for two Tylenol in the afternoon and want his back rubbed and a hot water bottle, that he would want more Tylenol after supper and another back rub and hot water bottle. I wrote down the times, because I thought that if there was a pattern to these backaches, it might help in the diagnosis. A few days later Scott started waking up around three or four in the morning because his back hurt. I'd give him more Tylenol and rub his back until he fell asleep again.

In August, Dr. Williams ordered complete back and chest X rays. I told him that I was determined that they had to do something about Scott's backaches. "But we can't treat until we know what we're treating," he said gently. "His tests haven't given us anything to go on. I'll call you if anything shows up on the X rays. Otherwise, come back in September."

Scott fell asleep as we were driving back to Fillmore, and I was free to let the tears roll down my cheeks. I was completely desperate. What had happened to my hopes of three months ago? What was God's will now?

Had I explained clearly enough how Scott felt? Did I make it clear to Dr. Williams that the attacks came like clockwork, that we could almost tell time by them? Did he understand how much pain Scott was in?

On Friday, August 24, I couldn't stand it any longer. I called Dr. Williams and told him that Scott's backaches were getting worse and that he had headaches and arm aches, too. He told me to come in on Monday. He would order a bone scan, since these symptoms seemed to be in the bone.

> I was cured. No more pain. No more aches. I was free from the chains of the hospital. For eight months I was the happiest person around. I did everything I wanted to. I was free from tests, shots, x-rays.
>
> Then about a week or two before school ended, I got a neckache. The next day I had it again. Soon I was having three or four a day. They got worse and worse. The pain moved from my neck down to the small of my back where it finally stayed. Now they would attack suddenly. I would be reading a book—then in a few seconds I would be crying in pain. Mostly I had them in the night. I couldn't sleep. I was getting weaker and weaker, pale and thin. Dr. Williams decided I should have a bone scan. Here is what it is—
>
> I got 2.0 microcuries of Polyphosphate Technetium intravenously. Then I had to wait four hours while the radioisotopes "soaked" into my bones. Then I was placed on a table under the scanner. The scanner is a very complicated machine. Actually, it's two machines. The part that takes the picture is circular, about two and a half feet in diameter. It is on an arm connected to a base. The other part is a computer about four feet

long with a screen where the radioisotopes can be seen. It also has switches, dials, numbers.

The radioisotopes gather where the bone is repairing itself where it has been damaged by disease. The scanner detects the radioisotopes and feeds the information into the computer. There are three screens on the computer and two have cameras fixed on them. The photograph comes out and is studied by the doctor.

I asked Scott what he'd like to do during the four hours he had to wait for the radioisotopes to soak into his bones. I had thought that he would probably want to visit one of the stores that sold military paraphernalia, but he decided he wanted to go to the Los Angeles County Museum of Natural History. It had a display on radiation that included a Geiger counter. When we walked by, the counter began to tick loudly.

Scott stopped. "Mom, I think I'm making it tick," he said.

"You do? Try it again. Walk over there and then come back," I suggested. When he went away, the Geiger counter slowed down; when he came back, it ticked faster and louder. We were experimenting with this when a man in a white coat introduced himself as Dr. Richards and asked if we were interested in the display.

"Oh, yes," Scott said happily. "Listen to the Geiger counter when I get near it."

Dr. Richards, rather skeptical, watched Scott walk toward the counter and heard it start ticking louder and faster. He asked Scott what kind of watch he was wearing and what he had in his pockets. Scott told the doctor that he thought it was the two microcuries of polyphosphate technetium that he had just been injected with that were affecting the counter. The doctor agreed that that was probably the cause. He took Scott into the booth where

the Geiger counter sat and moved the microphone over
Scott's body, which sent the counter into a frenzy of ticking.

When we returned to the hospital, Scott told Ken Day,
the radiotechnician in Nuclear Medicine, about his experience while Ken was supervising Scott's bone scan. This
was one of the few tests that was painless. It was even
interesting. Scott could see his bones on the screen as the
scanner moved over him. At one point, he said, "Look,
Mom, that's my femur." I could tell that Ken was startled.
I wasn't. Scott had spent hours and hours since his hospitalization a year and a half ago drawing his lymph
system, his blood system, and his bone structure. Ken
began to test him. He'd point at various bones as they
appeared on the screen and ask Scott to name them. Scott
got most of them right.

> **Ken Day did the scan. Afterwards, he gave me a pic-
> ture of my heart and my right hand. Then we went
> home and Mom got a phone call from Dr. Williams. All
> she said was that the bone scan showed something. Then
> that night Dad told me I was going to the hospital again.**

Ronnie and I had been at the store when Dr. Williams
called. There were no customers fortunately. When the
doctor told me that the scan had shown something, it was
almost more than I could bear. I put my head down on
the desk and cried.

"I just can't tell him, Ronnie," I sobbed. "I can't tell
him he has to go back to the hospital." "It's okay, honey,"
Ronnie told me gently. "It's okay. I'll tell him after work
tonight."

We had time for one special treat before Scott had to
go back to the hospital. We had tickets for the Hollywood
Bowl for September 1, when they would be playing
Tchaikovsky's *1812* Overture. Steven and Scott loved it.

The cannon and battle scene on the jacket of our record at home had first attracted their attention when they were about seven or eight and they had asked me to play it for them. They used to sit and draw battle pictures while it was playing.

When we moved to Fillmore, they discovered that the library lent phonograph records as well as books, and they checked out the whole Tchaikovsky repertoire and then went on to Strauss and Liszt, Bach and Beethoven and Prokofiev. But the *1812* was always special. It was the first "good" music that had made an impression on them, and we were all looking forward to the night at the Hollywood Bowl.

The traffic was backed up at the Bowl turnoff that night. It began to look as if we'd never get there. Ronnie let us out of the car and told us to walk the rest of the way and he'd join us when he could.

About halfway, Scott's back began to hurt. "Mom, I don't think I can make it," he gasped. "My back hurts so much." I gave him two Tylenol and said we'd rest until he felt better. Then a voice over the loudspeaker said no one would be admitted after the performance had started. Wildly I began to look for someone who might help me carry Scott, but then he said he thought he could walk some more. We finally made it. To me it was worth it just to see the boys' eager, intent faces as they listened to the music and their joyous excitement when the fireworks went off at the end.

On September 7, I got up about four in the morning to go to Childrens for an organ scan. This is a different scanning machine. It is smaller and takes about two or three hours for one side of the body. From 8:30 in the morning to 2:30 in the afternoon, I was under this slow machine.

Then the worst thing that I had feared, the thing that

occasionally gave me nightmares happened. Dr. Williams set a date for a bone biopsy and bone marrow test. On September 9, I was admitted to Childrens again. About ten on the tenth, a nurse came into my room and gave me a shot to relax me. I said goodbye to Mom and Dad.

I was in the operating room. Everything was green. There were two x-ray machines right by the operating table. This surgery was delicate. They look through the x-ray machine so they won't make a mistake and damage my spine I thought as I looked at the machines.

"Five milligrams pentothal," said the anesthesiologist. They put five in the I.V. Nothing. They put in a few more. I laughed. "Can't get me out, can you?" Then everything went blank. When I woke up, I was in the recovery room and everything I saw was double.

The next day Dr. Williams had some first-year medical students come in and ask me questions. They asked me about Hodgkin's, what I liked to do, what I thought about the hospital and stuff like that. Then they talked to Mom. After a while Mom came back in and said the med students told her they learned more about Hodgkin's talking with me than they could learn from books.

On September 14, I went to the doctor in Ventura for a spinal tap. Dr. Martin put me on a table and put a needle in my back to anesthetize the area. Then he drove a needle into my spinal cavity and let the spinal fluid drip out. When we got home, Dr. Martin phoned and said I had meningitis. I soon recovered, but I still was having backaches three or four times a day.

Two weeks later we went back to the clinic and Dr. Williams told me that Scott's biopsy had showed no Reed-Sternberg cells (the cells that confirm Hodgkin's), but that they did find other cells that are common in people

who have Hodgkin's. He said that he would order a neck
lymph node biopsy.

On October 8, I was admitted to Childrens again. I
had feared this, but thought it couldn't happen. Tomorrow I would have a biopsy of the left lymph node. That
night the intern came in with a tray of stuff. I noticed
an I.V. bottle on the tray.

"You're not going to put an I.V. in are you?" I asked.

"Yes," he said, "your blood count is low, so we have to
give you a transfusion.

"I'll use a size 19 needle," he told the nurse.

"Oh, no!" said the nurse. "That's far too big. Use a
21."

"Good grief," I thought. "He's a doctor and he
doesn't even know what size needle to use." I didn't
want a dummy who didn't know anything about needles
to touch me, much less work on me.

He took the long plastic tube out of its sterile case and
used a metal needle to pierce a hole through my skin
and vein and then pushed the plastic tube, which is
about two inches long, into my vein. The vein burst and
I had a gigantic raised bruise.

He tried again on the opposite side of my right arm
and got it in. But he tried to take blood from the same
arm and, of course, burst the vein again. I now had two
big raised bruises on my arm. I begged them to give me
a rest. They said they would come back later and try
again.

I huddled under my covers and tucked my arms as far
under me as I could, because I was afraid that if I fell
asleep they might sneak in and try to stick needles in me
and that, waking up, I might jerk my arms away and
hurt myself. The doctor and nurse came back later and
finally got the I.V. in. They put a bottle of glucose on to
run for a while. After a half hour they would replace it
with a bag of the blood I needed. Soon the blood was

slowly dripping into me. I dozed off occasionally, but I would wake myself up and keep watching the blood drip. All of a sudden I saw that the bag of blood was almost empty. I called the nurse and soon I was back on glucose.

That morning I didn't wake up because I never fell asleep. I was worried because it was almost time for me to be taken to surgery and my Mom and Dad had not arrived. The nurse started to roll me away to surgery. "No," I said. "Wait until my parents come." Just that moment they walked in. I said goodbye and was rolled to the same place I had been before.

"Put some pentothal in," said a doctor. They put some in. Then some more. And more. "I've gotten used to pentothal, huh?" I said. "Yeah," said the anesthesiologist. I fell asleep about two seconds after that.

All of a sudden I was awake, I tried to move my foot, but it was tied to the bed. I opened my eyes. Everything I saw was double because of the anesthetic. The nurse came over to take my blood pressure. She had four eyes, two noses and two mouths. When the anesthetic was worn off enough, I asked Mom where Dad was. She said he went shopping.

"For what?"

"Just something."

After a while Dad walked in. "I've got something for you," he said. It was a medal, the Purple Heart. I had started getting interested in medals and uniform insignia just before I went into the hospital in 1971. "Where'd you get that?" I asked. He gave me the name of the place. They were military suppliers. That night I wore my medal. The next morning I was discharged from the hospital. I stayed home for about a week or two and wore my medal all the time.

I was soon back in Los Angeles again. Dr. Williams told me I was to have treatments again. I've had three cycles of treatment, which now consists of Adriamycin.

Wait two weeks. Then vincristine and Cytoxan. Wait one week. Vincristine and Cytoxan again. Wait three weeks for Adriamycin and it starts all over again. The Adriamycin and the vincristine make me very sick now. I usually vomit as soon as I get one in me. Dr. Williams said my recovery had been very, very good and that I may be off treatment soon. I will not miss my treatments. But I will miss seeing my doctors.

This story is not complete. I could never write a complete story. There is too much pain, too many things I can remember. So many things. I could never write them all down.

Scott had missed the first weeks of seventh grade. And when he did go back to school, he found junior high very confusing. He had missed all the indoctrination and did not know what the different bells meant or where his rooms were. But slowly he became used to it.

His English teacher was very sympathetic. He was the one who encouraged Scott to write about his bone scan and the biopsy. Some of the things that Scott did not want to write about were perhaps too cruel for him to want to set down on paper.

One incident comes to my mind. He was late for one class. The teacher sent him to the office for a tardy slip. Fillmore Junior High School is a series of sprawling buildings and Scott's classroom was a good block from the office. He walked to the office, got his tardy slip, and walked back. Then the teacher made him stand beside his desk for ten minutes, punishment for being late.

When I picked Scott up for lunch, he was very pale and I could tell something was wrong. When he told me what had happened, I practically flew into the principal's office. He said he could not imagine anyone at the school allowing such a thing to happen. And he said it would not happen again. He transferred Scott to another class.

Scott was also very disturbed that the Adriamycin made his hair fall out. The drugs he had taken previously had caused some hair loss, but nothing like this. He refused to let me cut it because he wanted as much hair on his head as possible, but it looked very scraggly and strange. He was self-conscious about it and most of the time he wore one of the military hats from his collection. One afternoon in the store, a man looked at him and said, "My gosh, what's the matter with your hair?" Everyone turned and looked.

Scott was embarrassed, but he said quietly, "The drugs I take make it fall out." The man flushed and looked as if he wished there were a hole he could disappear into. Some of the kids at school were even crueler in their remarks. When Scott had to write an essay about man's inhumanity to man, he gave the example of when "somebody makes a cruel remark about my hair. It tears me apart. And I cannot do one thing about it unless I want to be plastered by some big bully."

But these things seemed trifles to me, if not to Scott, as hope surged back again. The Adriamycin took effect almost immediately. We could hardly believe how fast that drug worked. Scott's backaches stopped after the first treatment. Dr. Williams said he was "impressed" at how fast Scott's lymph nodes were going down. In January I took Scott to Los Angeles for another bone scan and it was perfectly normal. Even cautious Dr. Williams said things "look encouraging."

Every now and then Scott's treatments had to be postponed because he had a cold or an infection. His blood count would be too low. It depressed him knowing that as soon as he got over his bronchitis, or whatever, he would have to have a treatment. The new treatments made him vomit more than the previous ones. One night after a long bout of vomiting, Scott lay sprawled on the bathroom floor, leaning against the tub, too weak to get up.

White and sweating, he huddled into the big bath towel I had wrapped around him and waited for the next attack. Then he asked the question that I had asked so often.

"Why, Mom? Why, why, why?" he asked miserably.

There was no answer. I had asked God why myself a thousand times. Why was Scott captive of this relentless disease? Why did he have to suffer? When I finally helped my weary son back to his bed that night, I was so agonized for him that there was no question of my being able to sleep. I spent the few hours left before dawn by his bed watching over him.

Scott began to dread the treatments so much that the closer we got to the clinic, the "sicker" Scott would get. He would tell me that he thought he had a temperature or he felt "funny." When the doctor examined him, he would complain that he had a sore throat or was coming down with a cold or bronchitis. Sometimes he was right and they would not give him the treatment. Usually they would tell him that his white blood count was good and he had to have the treatment.

One beautiful spring day, we were driving to Ventura for his treatment. Dr. Williams had arranged for Scott to have some treatments in Ventura so we would not have to make the long trip to Los Angeles so often. Scott just sat looking out the window during the half-hour drive. When we got to the doctor's office, he said, "I'm not getting out."

I could not believe it. "Come on, Scott. You have to."

"No, Mom. I don't want any more treatments."

What could I say? I think I really wanted to tell him that he did not have to have any more treatments. I wanted to switch on the ignition, turn the car around, and head for home. But I was convinced that his treatments would cure him. He was getting better, I told myself. I couldn't let him give up.

"Scott, don't give up now," I pleaded. "I know how

awful it is. You've gone through so much. But don't give up. Please."

"I'm not getting out of the car." His face was set and determined.

I tried again. "We've been so proud of you. Remember when Dr. Williams said he couldn't have helped at all if it weren't for you? You're the one who had to do it. You've got to keep on being brave.

"Please," I begged him. "I love you. I want you to get well."

"Okay," Scott said in a low voice.

I got out, walked around, and opened his door. He just sat there. What would I do if he refused to get out? He sighed. And he got out. We walked into the building. Scott didn't look at me.

"Hi, Scott," Dr. Martin said with a big smile. "Why are you looking so glum today?" Scott didn't answer.

"He doesn't want his treatment," I said.

Dr. Martin did not understand the mood Scott was in and tried to cheer him up. "Come on," he said, "you're an old pro at this. Let me see that smile of yours."

It was impossible to tell him that he was going about things all wrong. I was afraid Scott would burst into tears. And if Scott didn't, I might. Fortunately the nurse sensed Scott's depression and said, "Why don't you come wait in the treatment room?" He followed her without a word. He lay there on the treatment table, his face turned toward the wall, and waited for the doctor. After his treatment, he vomited, and then we drove home again. Silently.

More and more often, Scott was sad. Once he was waiting on the treatment table when Dr. Fletcher, who, like Dr. Martin, was on the staff in Ventura, and often gave him his treatments there, took one look and asked, "What's the matter?"

"Nothing," Scott muttered without looking at him.

"Just tired of the whole thing? Is that it?" Dr. Fletcher asked in such an understanding voice that it brought tears to my eyes and I saw the nurse wipe away a few tears of her own.

"Yes," Scott said.

"Well, I don't blame you. I'll try my best, though, to give you the injection on the first try."

Scott stretched out his arm.

There were other days when Scott felt strong and he and Dr. Fletcher would chat and tease each other. "Boy, if the police ever get a look at your arms, they'll think you're an addict," Dr. Fletcher would tell him. "You'll be in the slammer for sure."

"I'll just say I got the stuff from you," Scott would retort.

The doctor laughed. "You know what I'll say? I'll say 'Scott who?' "

One day Dr. Martin told Scott he had a choice about his treatments.

"Oh yeah, what's the choice?" Scott asked.

"You can have your injection in any arm you choose," answered Dr. Martin.

Scott did not hesitate as he said, "I choose yours."

Just a year earlier, we had rejoiced when month after month Dr. Williams canceled Scott's treatments, but now when they were canceled, it triggered worries that often spiraled into black despair. Scott was happy when the doctor would say "no treatment today," but every time his blood count was too low for a treatment, I was plunged into the depths. This meant the disease was gaining. Early in April 1974 Dr. Williams said, "We'll try a few more courses of this present treatment."

"How much longer will I have to have them?" Scott asked.

"We'll just take two months at a time for now," the doctor said, glancing at me.

It was around this time that I learned that Richard, Scott's old roommate, was back in the hospital and not doing very well. We had not seen Joanne and Richard for a long time, because Scott had been getting most of his treatments in Ventura. I left Scott in the clinic to wait for his blood tests while I ran up to Four West to say hello to Joanne.

She and her mother were sitting by Richard's bed. I was shocked when I saw him. He was so wasted. It hurt to see him. He was lying there, not moving.

"Richard, Elaine's here to see you," Joanne said bending over him.

Richard moaned. I could tell that it was a tremendous effort. I told him I hoped he would feel better soon and then I left. Joanne followed me out and we talked for a few minutes. It was just a matter of time, she told me. Richard had almost died at Christmas. Now it was a matter of days, perhaps hours.

The day before, she said, she had made all the arrangements for Richard's funeral. "I planned the service and picked out the casket. It was the hardest day of my life," she told me. "It will take a miracle to save him. There are no more drugs they can use. They asked me if they could try a new drug. They said it was probably too late, but they wanted to see if there was any response. I told them to go ahead as long as it didn't hurt him."

"Perhaps this will turn out to be the miracle drug," I said.

She paid no attention to my remark, but went on to say that Dr. Williams had taken her aside. "He asked . . ." and she had to stop, her face working, until she regained control. "He asked if Richard's heart should stop, did I want them to try to revive him. I told him no. Richard's been through enough."

We stood looking at each other. Eyes of sadness. Eyes of despair. Of course it was over. I had known it the minute I saw Richard. He had fought and lost. And so had Joanne.

She asked how Scott was. I told her he was here for a treatment.

"Don't let him come up here," she said, putting her hand on my arm. "I wouldn't want him to see Richard now."

Two days later we were eating lunch by the pool when Joanne called. Richard had died that morning at four thirty, that loneliest hour. He had just slipped away quietly. He was twelve years old.

I stood holding the telephone for minutes after Joanne hung up. Tears in my eyes. Remembering the fun Scott and Richard had had together even when they were both feeling miserable. And the comfort they had been for each other in the hospital. Then I took Scott into our bedroom and told him.

Richard's death made a difference in Scott. I am sure he thought about it more than we ever knew. It was his first experience of a young friend dying. He never said a word about it, but I am sure that it made him wonder about his own future.

Chapter Eight

Scott hated and feared his treatments, but he liked all his doctors. And he loved Dr. Williams. We all did. He was a very special man. One time when Scott was in Childrens for surgery, Dr. Williams had said he would talk to Scott about the operation the night before. When we came back from having supper in the cafeteria, we were disappointed to hear that Dr. Williams had come by while we were away. The next morning Ronnie and I got to the hospital early to be with Scott before he was wheeled off to the operating room. Scott greeted us with, "Guess what? Dr. Williams came to see me last night!"

"He did! When?" I asked in some surprise since we had stayed until after ten.

"Around eleven. He told me just what they are going to do this morning. I felt a lot better after I talked with him."

Later that day I thanked Dr. Williams for seeing Scott the night before and told him that Scott had felt better after their chat. "We didn't expect you would come by so late," I said.

"I came earlier, but you had gone to eat," he said, "then I had to pick up my car from the garage where it was being repaired. When I got there, they told me it wasn't ready, so I came back to the hospital. But I discovered I didn't have any money for busfare, so I had to walk. That's why I was so late."

Another day I showed Dr. Williams one of Scott's drawings. Scott had shown himself as a soldier being attacked by syringes. Dr. Williams looked at it a long while, shaking his head. He called the picture "Scott's Shot Tree." "I can see myself in the hereafter," he said with a painful smile, "spread-eagled against a wall and all these kids coming at me with needles."

He is not one of those doctors who does not dare to get close to his patients. His patients love him and he returns their love. I remember seeing a three-year-old who had leukemia run up to him and say, "I want to give you a kiss." He picked her up and held her while she gave him a big, noisy kiss. Another day I watched him with a teenage girl and her mother. He took the girl's hand, winked at her mother, and said, "We're going to have a private talk, the two of us." He put his arm around the girl as they walked down the hall. I wondered what he was going to tell her—a new treatment, surgery, a bad blood count. My heart went out to both doctor and patient, and I thought of the tremendous emotional toll his work must take of him.

To Scott, it was as if Dr. Williams were another grandfather. He always brought something along to show him— a book he was reading, a medal he had just acquired, a fossil he had found in the hills. Once he brought the head of a little mouse that Steven had mounted the way people mount moose heads—only this was a sweet little mouse that had a very surprised expression as if to say, "What am I doing here?"

It was very seldom that Dr. Williams did not hop up on the examining table after he had finished checking Scott and sit there with his arm around him while they talked

for a few minutes. One day Scott brought his tape recorder and taped his session with Dr. Williams. This ex-
cerpt gives an idea of the warmth and thoughtfulness of
the man.

DR. WILLIAMS:	What's this? (*Scott was showing him some snapshots of Steven and an owl.*)
SCOTT:	It's a Tito Alba Pratincola.
DR. WILLIAMS:	Now, tell me, Scott, where is this?
SCOTT:	This is up Sespe. And that's me. (*Scott spread out snapshots of himself and Steven hiking along Sespe Creek.*)
DR. WILLIAMS:	Is that the one that ran wild when they had the flood?
SCOTT:	Yes.
DR. WILLIAMS:	Are there any trout in there?
SCOTT:	Oh, yeah, lots of them.
DR. WILLIAMS:	How do you get to Sespe? Can you go camping there?
SCOTT:	Sure. Once you get to Fillmore, drive all the way up to the end and start hiking. You take Grand Avenue to the end.
DR. WILLIAMS:	I see. That'll be the jumping-off point. It's quite primitive up there, isn't it?
SCOTT:	Once you get past a few miles from Devil's Gate, you don't see too many people. And when you get off into the side creeks like Pine Creek, then you see hardly anybody.

A pause while Dr. Williams looks at Scott's chart.

SCOTT:	How's my blood count?
DR. WILLIAMS:	Your white count still seems to be staying down a little.
SCOTT:	Are you going to give me my shot?
DR. WILLIAMS:	Well, we decided to hold off your shots be-cause of your white count. I think what it means is that you're still showing the effects of the Adriamycin.

SCOTT (*happily*):   So I don't get any shot?

> *Dr. Williams smiles and starts examining Scott.*

DR. WILLIAMS: Well, that looks good, Scott.

ME: How long do the effects of the Adriamycin usually last?

DR. WILLIAMS: Usually two to three weeks. With some, it's been three weeks. With him having had a lot of treatment in the past, I think that he may have the effects a little longer. . . . Okay, get dressed, Scott. You know, I think what we should maybe do for next week is get a count in Ventura. That way we can make a decision after we see if it's up. I'd like to see it going up instead of down.

ME: Does this make a difference in the Cytoxan working?

DR. WILLIAMS: Well, the vincristine doesn't run down the white count. It's the Cytoxan and Adriamycin that are knocking down his count. His weight is up a little now.

SCOTT (*encouraged*):   Oh.

ME: He's been feeling better.

DR. WILLIAMS: So I think it's probably the effects of his previous treatment and he's a little sensitive to the drugs. (*Turning to Scott.*) You've been feeling better?

SCOTT: Yes, I've been feeling real good this week. (*Pause.*) Dr. Williams, I wanted to ask you. You teach students . . .

DR. WILLIAMS: Yeah.

SCOTT: Are you a professor?

DR. WILLIAMS: Yep.

SCOTT: When do you teach them?

DR. WILLIAMS: Well, I'm with them every Tuesday morning. And Thursday afternoon.

SCOTT: How long have you been in hematology?

DR. WILLIAMS: Oh, um, fifteen years. Longer than you've been around.

SCOTT: How does it work? You're with Childrens and
                    the university?

DR. WILLIAMS: Actually, all of us have appointments in the
                    department. The full-time staff at Childrens
                    are professors at USC. We teach courses in
                    hematology, teach the interns and the medical
                    students. I'm also involved in a special course
                    where we teach the first-year medical students
                    how to take a history and give a physical. We
                    start that the first week they're in school.

SCOTT: Neat!

DR. WILLIAMS: We try to teach them the humanity of it so
                    they don't get lost in the blood counts and
                    other things. . . . (*He turns away to the desk.*)
                    I'll put a tentative appointment down for
                    next week if your blood count goes up.

SCOTT: I hope you're able to come up sometime and
                    see the Sespe.

DR. WILLIAMS: I'd like that. We're going to try and do a little
                    camping this summer.

According to Dr. Williams's instructions, Scott had a
blood test in Ventura the next week. His white blood
count was up enough so he could resume his treatments.

Chapter Nine

DESPITE his frequent absences, Scott finished seventh grade with flying colors, making the honor roll. He looked forward to a long summer devoted to camping, hiking, and following his many interests. "I can hardly wait for you to get back," he wrote to one of his friends. "We'll hike all over the hills and up the creeks, down the canyons and past the rattlesnakes. We'll swim for days straight in our pool and have a great time." That was the life Scott longed for. And the few times that summer that he felt well enough to go on a short hike, he enjoyed every hot, sweaty moment of it. But it turned out to be a summer of one disappointment after another.

The Adriamycin was taking its toll. After his June 14 injection, his blood counts were too low to continue his treatments. He had a blood test every week, and on July 3 his count was down to 650. A healthy white blood count is 5000 to 10,000. And Scott felt miserable. He had cut his little finger, just a small cut, the kind you'd never think anything of, probably not even bother to do anything about except wash it and let the air get at it. But Scott had no resistance to infection. Soon there was an angry red streak up his arm. At the same time he developed a gum infection and his jaw was swollen.

Both infections responded to penicillin, but not in time for Scott to enjoy the Fourth of July. We had planned a big party and had a lot of fireworks to set off after dark. But Scott was so dragged down by his infections that he spent the day on the couch in the living room while his friends were out in the backyard splashing and swimming and playing games in the pool. He set off a few firecrackers when the sun went down, but he was too tired to enjoy it. I thought of previous Fourths when he and Steven had run around waving sparklers in the dark and helping Ronnie set off the big rockets. But this year, Scott simply lit a few red firecrackers and tossed them into the air and then he was exhausted.

The following week in Los Angeles, Dr. Williams told him to keep getting the weekly blood tests in Ventura until he came back to Childrens in August. "We'll discuss a new drug program then," he said. For the time being Scott's blood count was far too low for him to have his treatment. The count started going up once Scott was off the treatment. He began to feel better, so much better that he was sure he'd be able to go to our church's annual camp for junior high schoolers, a week at Hume Lake. He and Steven were looking forward to it excitedly, but the day before they were to leave, Scott had his weekly blood test. It was low. Much too low.

"You mean I can't go to camp?" Scott asked.

"It just wouldn't be wise, Scott," Dr. Martin said.

Scott nodded. On the way home he said quietly, "I'm tired, Mom. I understand why Dr. Martin said no."

The next morning after I drove Steven to the bus and waved him off with the other boys, I drove through the orange groves and stopped where no one could see me. I had to be alone with my tears. I kept thinking that this trip Steven was making alone was a kind of preparation for a future time when Steven would always have to go places without Scott.

I began dreading any special event that Scott looked forward to—a picnic, a hike, a cookout, a party. He had to miss so many of them. His blood count would be too low. He would be tired. Or he would have a sore throat or an infection. I wanted him to have all the good times he could, but he was too weak to do most of the things that he wanted to do that summer.

In August Dr. Williams asked all four of us to come to Childrens so they could take blood samples. Earlier in the summer Dr. Williams had gone to Seattle to discuss Scott's case with doctors at the medical center there who had done some pioneering work in bone-marrow transplants. These transplants had been performed only on leukemia patients, not on anyone with Hodgkin's. Dr. Williams was particularly interested because the researchers had discovered that the best results were obtained when the transplants were from one identical twin to another, and he wanted to see if the procedure might help Scott. He explained that they gave high dosages of radiation and drugs to kill off all the cells in the patient's bone marrow and then injected healthy bone marrow from the donor. Now he wanted blood samples from the four of us to send to Seattle.

The samples were packed in dry ice and then rushed by helicopter to a plane that would deliver them to Seattle. I was deeply thankful that there were still possible cures for Scott, that we had not exhausted every resource. I kept thinking of what Joanne had told me about Richard. "There are no more drugs they can use," she had said sadly. But there was this new procedure for Scott. Perhaps this would be it. I was excited and hopeful about the bone-marrow transplant, even though Dr. Williams had made it clear to Ronnie and me that they either cured— or killed.

Steven had assured us that he was willing to give his bone marrow to help Scott. Scott, however, was not very enthusiastic about the idea of more surgery. He had been hurt too often. But Dr. Williams said that there was no need to decide anything yet. "Let's wait and not think too much about it," he said, "until I hear from Seattle. We'll keep this as our ace in the hole." There would be plenty of time for us to think about it carefully before we had to make the final decisions. If we decided to go ahead with it, we would have to take both boys to Seattle and plan to stay there for at least a month. And Scott would have to be in good shape. The results of the transplants were better when the patient was in good health. We had no idea that Scott would never be strong enough to make this operation feasible.

They stopped giving me Adriamycin, which was doing more harm than good. It causes unhealthy side effects after it builds up in the body, so Dr. Williams decided I had had enough and took me off. When I went to see the doctor on August 2, they all were getting together to decide which treatment to put me on now. The choices: chemotherapy with vincristine and Cytoxan, radiation, a bone marrow transplant.

The latter is a very new operation and there is a lot to be known about it. I would much rather have the chemotherapy, for the bone marrow transplant is so new. It consists of a few very heavy doses of vincristine and Cytoxan and total body irradiation to knock out all my bone marrow completely. Then I would get some bone marrow from my brother. And then I would be free of disease and live happily ever after. *If* the transplant would take. If not—poor, poor me.

As I sit here watching the rain, listening to the last notes of Tchaikovsky's Sixth Symphony, I wonder what is in store for me. I don't really care. I just thank God for what He has done and appreciate every precious second of life.

There were moments, however, that were hard to appreciate. Times like the day when Scott asked the doctor, "Can I have a finger stick today when they take the blood for my test? They don't have to take it from my arm, do they?"

"Sure, tell them to take it from your finger," the doctor said. "We don't need that much blood today."

This was a great relief. The finger stick took longer, but it was much easier on Scott. It almost always took two or three, sometimes four painful probes before the technicians could find a vein in his arm. There was a new technician in the lab that day, young and very pretty.

"Let me see your arm, Scott," she said after reading the lab order for the blood test.

"Can't you take it from my finger?" he asked.

"It's much easier to take it from your arm," she said and grasped Scott's wrist as she rolled up his sleeve.

Scott looked at me. "Mom, the doctor said I could have a finger stick."

"It hurts worse to have your finger stuck than a quick needle jab," the pretty girl said. She was already searching his arm for a vein.

"The doctor told him he could have a finger stick," I said, wondering if I should tell her how rare a "quick needle jab" was for Scott.

"Well, all right," she said impatiently, "I'll take it from your finger. But only babies have finger sticks." Scott sat quietly as she drew the blood from his finger. I was angry. At the same time, I was afraid to say anything, not afraid of the technician, but simply of flying off the handle in front of Scott. I thought it would upset him. The more I thought about the episode, the madder I got. When I told Ronnie about it, he was angry with me for letting that girl insult Scott. He said I should have complained to the doctor immediately.

The next time I took Scott for a blood test, I told the doctor what had happened. He picked up the telephone immediately and asked for the head of the lab. "Scott was in the lab for a CBC the other day," he said, "and one of the technicians called him a baby for wanting a finger stick.

"We need to save his veins for his chemotherapy treatments. From now on, unless I specify otherwise, I want only finger sticks for Scott."

I started to apologize for complaining, but he said quite sharply, "If you don't stick up for your own child, who will? Don't ever be afraid to make a complaint."

Chapter Ten

IT WAS back-to-school time again, always a hard anniversary. The memory of that autumn three years ago when Scott first complained that it hurt to swallow was always sharper in September. He had been starting fifth grade then, an eager, boisterous little boy; now he was starting the eighth grade. He had not grown perceptibly in those three years. The drugs, as Dr. Williams had warned us, had arrested his development. He looked much younger than thirteen going on fourteen, but his eyes were ageless. Sometimes I looked into Scott's eyes and saw such compassion, such understanding, that I would have to turn away to conceal my tears. At times, they were still a little boy's eyes, full of wonder, delight, and mischief; other times they were puzzled and clouded by pain. But more and more, those brown eyes looked out on the world with a gaze of luminous sympathy, a sympathy I knew was born of pain and his inner struggle for acceptance of God's will.

What would become of my son? I still kept telling myself that the doctors had been wrong. He had lived one more year than they had thought he would. There was hope in this. And more hope in the fact that Scott was able to do so many things. He had wanted to be in the band again this year, but the marching was just too much for him, so he settled for playing the kettledrum in the school orchestra instead. He threw himself into all the school activities, attended the football games and the Friday-night dances. The fact that most of the girls were almost a foot taller than he was didn't bother him in the least. He danced every dance until he got tired.

He was so eager to participate in everything that he asked Dr. Williams if he could change his treatment day so he wouldn't miss so much school. Dr. Williams worked out a compromise that made Scott happy. He would have his checkup twice a month at Childrens on Fridays and then have his treatments in Ventura on Saturdays. This way he could take part in all the Friday-night events and not have to miss any school.

Scott had shown Dr. Williams some of the material he had written for school about his illness and his hospital experiences. That fall, Dr. Williams asked Scott if he could use some of Scott's reports for a lecture he was going to give in San Francisco. Scott delightedly gave his permission. The doctor also asked if he and Steven would write about their reactions to his illness. Of course they would. They would have done anything he asked. Steven wrote:

I feel sorry for my brother. He comes home from the hospital looking like a zombie. He doesn't eat as much and I am a mite taller and a lot heavier. I remember the first time they called and said he might have one of a number of undesirable diseases. I didn't know how serious it was, but I thought it was short term. I felt somewhat insecure those weeks, because I lived at my grandparents and with friends. I hardly ever saw Mom. I was relieved when he came home. He looked like a white sheet—thirty-one pounds with zero disease resistance.

The only thing that affects me is that I have had to become more independent. Sometimes Scott gets mad at small things, but who cares? I have found that my parents love me just the same, but they do things for him because of all this. He does seem to be stubborn. He must have what he wants. He argues and talks back to everyone. If things aren't perfect, he has to make them that way. I give in sometimes. I can accept something else or improvise. And I don't argue much either.

Scott wrote:

I'm glad they have these medicines to cure Hodgkin's disease, but I don't like their side effects. I wish the injections could be spaced farther apart. By the time I really get to feeling good, it's time for more shots. If they were spaced farther apart, I would have time for myself. It seems as if doctors sometimes don't take into consideration that people my age like time to follow their interests.

I can see that getting well comes first, but then again, if I'm going to be on this treatment for a while, most likely a few years, I'd rather have my injections spaced so that I'd have more time for myself and be on the program for twice the time instead of not feeling well for half the time.

Sometimes I get depressed. I wish that I could just run away, get away from all this medicine. I just want it to stop for a while, to rest from it all. But I don't stay depressed for long. I know that everything is going well. There are always people worse off than me and they make it. So I can too. I know that all will go well. I am very lucky to have a disease that can be cured. I pray that others might be as lucky.

Scott was writing more these days. He seemed to have a great deal that he wanted to get down on paper. After he had described his feelings about his illness for Dr. Williams, he started a diary.

> November 22, 1974—It is clear with a few fluffy white clouds over San Cayetano. The cool breeze and sunshine, the crystal clear sky have a gloomy note for I am now riding to Ventura to get my shot. What a terrible thing to have to get on a beautiful day like this. I'll miss the football game tonight. That makes me mad. I feel like I want to get away. I want to run from the shot. I want to hide. I need a rest just for a while. It's as if a big monster is trying to consume me, to engulf me. I try to run, but there is no way. I'm trapped.
>
> November 23, 1974—When I stand in the sun, it's warm with the wind wiping off the excess sunshine. It's the day after my shot. This morning I got up, ate a little Cream of Wheat and then rested on the sofa, finally falling asleep about one o'clock for almost an hour. I woke up, had lunch and now I'm writing this.
>
> November 24, 1974—Went to Frank Putnam's fourteenth birthday party. We went to a miniature golfing place in Ventura. I came in fourth among seven people.
>
> November 28, 1974—Today is Thanksgiving. We had Thanksgiving at our house this year with Grandma Roma, Grandma and Grandpa McMaster, Mark, Kym, Phyllis and Aunt Hazel. I didn't eat much turkey though. I wasn't very hungry this year.
>
> November 29, 1974—We are at the STOP sign on the way up to the pines near San Cayetano. It looks like a bear has torn the sign up (1:35 p.m.) At the end of the hike, I'm very tired. Found some feathers from a female Tito Alba Pratincola's right wing. It was a very nice hike. A few times I thought I wouldn't make it. We didn't get all the way to the pines, but Mom thought it was a great achievement for me. I'm plenty tired (4 p.m.)

That last entry referred to a hike that Steven and Scott and their friend Jeff Fauver had made to the pine forest in the foothills of San Cayetano. They had been planning it for a long time and Scott was finally strong enough to make it. Since the area was too remote for them to hike into alone, I went along with them. I got permission from the Forest Service to drive up the dirt road that led to the mountain as far as the first gate. Normally this road is off bounds to everyone except the Forest Service, but when I explained that Scott had limited reserves of energy, they gave permission.

We had not gone far when Scott sat down saying he did not think he could go any farther. We stopped to let him rest, and then I suggested that Steven and Jeff go ahead while Scott and I followed at a slower pace. I suspected that Scott would not be able to complete the six-and-a-half-mile hike along a trail that wound steadily upward, but they all had looked forward to the outing so much that I did not want to turn back unless we had to. Scott looked tired already, but we walked on slowly. Steven and Jeff went ahead and were soon out of sight.

And then I began to worry. There were mountain lions and bobcats and bears in this area. What would Jeff and Steven do if they ran into one of them? But then at a turn in the trail, there were Steven and Jeff waiting for us. We went on that way. Scott and I would rest, then walk.

At one rest stop, I peeled an orange. Then I thought—this is going to attract bears. And the bears will kill the boys to get more food. Suddenly I was cold—despite the temperature in the nineties.

"Boys, we'd better start back. It'll be dark soon."

Steven and Jeff begged me to let them go on as far as the pine forest. Scott said, "They'd be there by now if they hadn't had to wait for me all the time. We can stay here and they can go on." I agreed. But the moment Steven and Jeff were out of sight, I began worrying again.

We were on the shady side of the mountain, and they were going deeper and deeper into the wilderness.

"Come on, Scott," I said, "we've got to get them."

"Mom, I can't. I'm tired."

"Then you stay here and I'll go." I started running up the trail. Then I thought— How can I leave Scott alone for the bears to eat? So I went back. Scott was sitting under the tree where I'd left him, listening to Beethoven's *Pastoral* on his tape recorder. I told him to follow me up the trail at his own pace. "Just answer me when I call," I said. "That's all I want—you near enough so I can hear you."

Scott laughed. "The bears won't bother me. I don't have enough meat on me."

I caught up with Steven and Jeff a half mile up the trail. This time I insisted that we all turn back.

One thing that Scott did not put in his diary was the time he got "arrested" for driving without a license. Well, not really. But that's the way we used to tease him about the incident. Scott had been much more interested in the 1934 Ford that Ronnie had restored than Steven, so Ronnie had said it could be Scott's when he was sixteen. Steven could have the pickup that Ronnie was also putting in shape, which was fine with Steven because he could use it for camping trips.

We taught both boys to drive on the little private roads that crisscrossed the orchards around Fillmore. One afternoon they and their friend Frank Putnam asked me to take them out and let them drive the '34. I let them take turns going around the blocks of orchards. Scott was so short that he could barely peer over the steering wheel. We passed some boys he knew, and when they spotted Scott behind the wheel, they doubled up in laughter. I told Scott to make a left. He waited too late, so I said,

"Okay, take the next left," without realizing that this would take us onto a two-lane highway instead of a private orchard road. I told him to take the next right so we could get back into the orchards.

"There's a cop behind us," Frank said suddenly.

"Sure," I said. Frank liked to play the clown and this was typical of his sense of humor.

"I'm not kidding," he said. Then with panic, he said, "He's got his light on!"

And he did.

"What shall I do?" Scott asked.

"You've got to pull over and stop. No, not now! There's a ditch there. And you can't stop in the middle of the road."

"Well, what'll I do?" he said, flustered, driving along about ten miles an hour.

"Put your hand out and signal that you're slowing down so he'll know you're going to stop." He finally reached a place wide enough to stop. The policeman came up to the car and asked Scott for his license. Scott looked almost too scared to speak, so I answered, "He doesn't have a license, sir."

"May I see your license then."

"How old are you?" he asked Scott.

"Almost fourteen."

"That's not even old enough for a permit," he scolded both of us, then walked behind the car to write out the ticket. I wanted to jump out and tell him how much this funny old car meant to Scott and that chances were he would never get to be old enough to have a learner's permit, let alone a license. But I reminded myself how determined Ronnie and I were that Scott lead a normal life—and that meant no favors.

The policeman returned my license, gave me the ticket, and told Scott, "Now, don't bug your mother to let you go driving until you have your permit." One shook-up mother drove three scared boys home—very slowly.

> **December 13, 1974—I am in the Hemo Clinic. I am depressed. I have to get my shot. It is a nice day in Fillmore—warm, clear and windy. Here in the city it is very smoggy. I don't want to get my shot. I felt like running away last night so I wouldn't have to get it.**
>
> **December 14, 1974—Sat around all day in bed and on sofa. Didn't feel too good, but not too bad.**
>
> **December 15, 1974—Went to get a Christmas tree. We cut it from a tree place in Santa Paula. I feel pretty good today, but not perfect. Mom and Steve decorated the tree while I was sleeping. So what? I am tired.**
>
> **December 19, 1974—Depressed at prospect of going to get injection tomorrow.**

On December 23, Scott woke up with a sore throat. On Christmas Eve, he developed a cough. And on Christmas morning, he woke with a high fever. Much as I hated to call on Christmas, I telephoned Dr. Martin who told me to bring Scott to Ventura as soon as possible. We drove right over and he gave Scott an antibiotic.

By New Year's Eve, Scott was feeling better. At midnight Ronnie and I watched the boys setting off fireworks to welcome the New Year. I looked up into the cold, starry sky and prayed— Please God, let 1975 be the year. I felt three other silent prayers joining mine.

> **January 6, 1975—Went to school and to the store after school. I'm starting to gain weight—a whole 64 pounds I weigh. Starting to feel pretty good too.**
>
> **January 8, 1975—Sunset a beautiful blue, a cross between purple and sky blue, a dark, but glowing sky blue. It almost describes my feelings sometimes—gloomy, but happy. A glowing alive feeling.**

January 9, 1975—The thought of tomorrow, the trip to Los Angeles, my treatment and the terrible sickness after it. Oh, the torment! Tomorrow, tomorrow . . .

Dr. Williams no sooner walked into the examining room on January 10 than Scott asked, "Do I have to get my treatment today? My birthday is Monday and I don't want to be sick on it. It's not fair to be sick on my birthday."

"Well, Scott, let's see what we can do," the doctor said as he looked over Scott's test results. "Hmmm. Your X rays are normal. In fact, they are the best ever. I think that we can try one extra week between treatments now—and later maybe two extra weeks. What you can do is get your next two treatments in Ventura, then come back here February twenty-first. How's that sound?"

"Great," Scott exclaimed. No one could have given him a better birthday present.

Scott and Steven celebrated their fourteenth birthday playing miniature golf with some of their friends and then stopping at McDonald's for hamburgers and milk shakes. A few days later, Ronnie and I took them to Big Bear for three days of fun in the snow. We went ice skating—a first for the boys—rode horses along snow-covered trails and went sledding on the hills. Scott tired easily, but to our delight he was able to do everything. Both boys had a wonderful time.

I missed my talks with Joanne when I took Scott to the clinic these days. There were other women there whom I liked, but Joanne and I had been especially close. And I was not certain that I wanted to be that intimate with another woman whose child had cancer. It had been so heart-wrenching when Richard died. I understood far better now what lay behind the seeming brusqueness and coldness of many of the hospital staff. It was the result of seeing too many children die. It was their defense against heartbreak. I learned not to make judgments. I came to understand that almost everyone at the hospital and clinic was truly dedicated. And everyone was human. We all protect ourselves against pain in our own way.

My way was not getting close to any other mothers and children after Joanne and Richard. But then I met Carolyn and Scott LaPorte. They came from Oxnard, which is close to Ventura, and I discovered that her Scott, who was five, was also a patient of Dr. Martin and Dr. Williams. He was in remission from neuroblastoma, a cancer of the nervous system that is usually fatal in young children. "We believe differently from some people," Carolyn told me. "I don't believe it is just a remission. I believe Scott is healed."

Little Scott looked and acted healthy when he was at the clinic. But then the tumor came back. He was given radiation and was in and out of the hospital for treatments and transfusions. As a result I did not see Carolyn for several weeks. Then I ran into her one day in Ventura. She told me that they would be at the clinic on Friday when Scott and I would be there.

"My Scott looks pretty bad now," Carolyn said. "He's lost a lot of weight because of the radiation. We don't even wait in the waiting room anymore. The nurses always take us straight into an examining room because he's so weak.

"I just wanted you to know," she said, "so you won't be too shocked if you do see him."

Nothing could have prepared me for the change in her little boy. I had to leave the room after a few minutes so I wouldn't cry in front of him. Carolyn caught up with me in the hall and put her arm around me. "I know that God can still cure him," she told me. "I'm not giving up yet," comforting me when I should have been comforting her. "But I don't think your Scott should see him," she said. And I agreed.

But one of the clinic volunteers told me that Scott had seen little Scott while he was getting one of his tests and that she thought it had upset him. All he said to me at the time though was, "I saw Scott."

A few nights later, Scott and Aunt Hazel were watching a religious program on TV that encouraged people to call in with their prayer requests. Scott called in a request for prayers for Scott LaPorte. But our prayers were not enough to save him. Carolyn called me the first day of February and said, "Scott went home to heaven this morning."

Scott and I grieved for both of them. There was a change in Scott that winter, imperceptible at the time, but as I look back on it, a very definite change. His attitude toward his illness and his treatments changed. It was evident in his diary entries and his writings. There was a new sadness and despair—even when he was feeling pretty good. Sometimes it was hard to remember that "feeling good" for Scott at this time was what most of us would call "feeling rotten."

We arrived at the hospital at eleven. I walked in, threw my empty Pepsi can into a trash can, went to the escalator, stepped off at the second floor, went to the lab, handed in my slip and card, went into the waiting room —and waited.

While I was waiting, I started thinking. "I've got to get out of here," I thought. "I hate this place. A closed room with a bunch of sick kids and stale air. I don't belong here. I should be in Fillmore, with my friends, in school."

An electrical sounding voice called, "Scott Ipswitch to the lab, please." I was glad to leave the room filled with rambunctious kids throwing blocks, overturning chairs, yelling, screaming, crying.

Why must I suffer? I must get away from it. Run! Hide! Go from the sterile, saline, white aseptic hospital, the smoggy city. I must leave it before it kills me. I must go into the fresh green grass with fresh cool droplets of dew sparkling in the light of early morning, breaking and beaming down from the billowing, majestic, raw clouds. The towering mountains. The majestic deer. Rocks. The ever-rushing stream, slipping through the smooth, clean rocks.

We had become so accustomed to Scott's feeling bad that when he said he felt better, we almost felt as if he were well. In a way, we had become blinded through familiarity to the implacable inroads of his disease, with the result that sometimes we expected too much from him. And when we realized it, we felt awful. Looking back, though, I would have done the same things again. Our mistakes were loving ones and made in an effort to give him a normal life.

Ronnie and I had always told the boys that, when they were fourteen, their allowances would stop and they would have to earn their own spending money. There were plenty of ways to earn that money—mowing the lawn and doing yard work, cleaning the pool, helping out in the store. Both boys liked the idea of earning their own money. And after their fourteenth birthday, we assigned each of them weekly chores that must be done. But then Steven began to feel that Scott was not doing his share. It was true. Scott did not work as hard as Steven. Part of it was just normal adolescent goofing off and taking advantage of not feeling well. But most of it was that he just did not have the strength. It became evident that even the lightest yard work was too exhausting for Scott on a regular basis. There were days when he could manage—and other days when Steven would have to do his share as well as his own. They had a number of fights about this.

Ronnie and I decided that Steven would work in the yard and clean the pool and Scott would work at the store where he could do most things sitting down. This was fine with Steven, who much preferred being outside. Scott ran up sales and made change, wrapped packages, and helped us straighten up the stockroom out back.

There were times when I would be busy with customers and wonder what took Scott so long to put half a dozen shoe boxes away. Later I was to discover that our stockroom was a treasury of little drawings and messages hidden away in unexpected spots. We discovered them one at a time—a small signboard with the legend Private —No Admittance over a keyhole. Beside a knothole was an inscription, Frankenstein lives here. And there were several tiny mice with captions reading, I was here or Scott was here. This solved the mystery of Scott's dawdling out back.

I would have preferred that Scott not have to do any chores and save his energy for the things he liked to do, but Dr. Williams said, "You know, Elaine, it wouldn't be fair to Steven. Or Scott. The best thing is to treat both boys the same and expect them to do their share. Just treat Scott normally." He was right, of course, but for a time that winter it seemed that whenever there was something special Scott wanted to do, he would be too sick or too weak. That just did not seem right.

One morning just after Easter we awoke early to the sound of bleating and looked up to find the hills speckled with sheep. The boys rushed home from school that afternoon to get their water canteens and then climb into the hills to see the sheep close to. The young Spanish

shepherd—his name was Pleno—offered them bread and
cheese and wine and showed them how the sheep dogs
helped him. After that, enchanted by the young shepherd
and his stories of his nomadic life with his flocks, they
went up every day after school, taking Pleno oranges and
Cokes and film for his camera.

When it was time for Pleno to move the sheep on to
new grazing grounds, the boys wanted to hike up and say
good-bye, but Scott had had a treatment the day before
and was pretty weak, even though the treatments did not
knock him out quite so much as they used to. I wanted
him to stay home and rest, but he wanted to go so much
that Ronnie drove the boys as close to the hill as he could
and then stayed by the car and watched them through his
binoculars. Scott had promised to signal if he got too
tired and needed help.

Ronnie came home a little later. "Scott just won't give
in," he said, his voice husky with emotion. He told me
that Steven had climbed halfway up the hill in the time it
took Scott to go a few yards. Scott would walk as far as he
could, then rest, then start again. When he got halfway
up, he waved to Ronnie and indicated that Ronnie
should not wait any longer.

The treatments seemed to be helping, and when Jim
Fauver, Jeff's father, planned a camping trip along the
Agua Blanca Creek, Scott insisted that he was strong
enough to go along. They planned to leave Friday, camp
out that night, hike all day Saturday, camp out Saturday
night, then hike home on Sunday.

Friday afternoon I drove the campers up the dusty oil
road to Squaw Flat, where they would start hiking. It is a
good hour's drive, and we were well into the wilderness
at the end. Webb had come along to see the boys off and
keep me company on the drive back home over the steep
and tortuously twisting road.

I tried to smile and not show my worry. The night before, Ronnie had told me impatiently, "Quit worrying. Jim will take good care of Scott. If anything happens to him, Jim will carry him out on his back if necessary."

"What if something happens to Jim?"

Ronnie sighed. "Will you just quit worrying?"

"Are you sure you want to go?" I asked Scott for the twentieth time.

"Yeah, Mom, I'm sure. I can make it. Quit worrying."

But I couldn't. Now that we were here at Squaw Flat, as far into the wilderness as the Forest Service permits cars to go, I asked Webb if he'd mind if we walked part of the way up the trail. We stayed with Jim and the boys until the first rest stop. I took some pictures and then Webb, who was leaning against a rock looking through his binoculars, said, "Take a look." He handed the glasses to Scott.

"Condors!" Scott exclaimed. Two condors were circling the hill in front of us—giant birds with wingspans that must have been at least seven or eight feet. We were close to the Sespe Condor Sanctuary, but even so, two condors wheeling and circling majestically were a rare sight.

When the condors disappeared, the boys began looking for fossils. Soon I was loaded with rocks to take home. As I was saying good-bye, Webb asked Steven, who was wearing a felt Stetson, "You got any hats besides that one?"

Steven shook his head. "Well," Webb said, "that thing's gonna bump against the frame of your backpack and really give you hell."

Steven just grunted an acknowledgment, but when he got home, he told me, "Webb was right. That hat was a pain."

Then Webb turned his attention to Scott. He pulled a big plastic garbage bag out of his shirt and gave it to him.

"Scott, if you have to cross the river and it's over your head, put your pack and clothes in this bag. Fill it with air and float it across. That way you'll have dry clothes when you reach the other side."

One of my big worries had been the Narrows, one of the hazards on the Agua Blanca trail. The sides of the canyon are straight up and down along the Narrows, high, sheer cliffs. If the water was high, you had to swim across or hike several miles up and around the area. I had worried about their swimming across and having no dry clothing to put on afterward and Scott getting cold. Thanks to Webb, I could forget about that worry.

Steven, who has his own writing talent and style, wrote about the trip later. I think he captured the special quality of their wilderness experience:

> The road up the hills was a rough one, steep and hot, but we managed to get up it with no problems. We rested a few times on the way up and when we got to the top took a long rest. We enjoyed the fresh smell of the junipers and sage. Jeff and I went down the trail to see if we could reach Cow Spring. About five minutes after we started, Jeff unknowingly put his foot an inch from a rattler's head.
>
> "There's a snake right by you, Jeff!" I yelled.
>
> Jeff looked around a bit and didn't move. He saw no snake. I picked up a rock and yelled "By your foot, damnit!" and he jumped out of the way so I could cream the snake.
>
> Soon after the four of us had gone over the pass near Bucksnort, we arrived in a flatter, wider valley. It sticks in my memory as a most beautiful area. Surrounded by chaparral and pine-covered mountains. Then we discovered to our delight a cool looking glade of pines in a canyon not very far away. Below we could see Agua Blanca and to the north rose Cobblestone Mountain (6,700 feet). We signed a register box and took off.

I'm holding Steven the day
after he was released from
the hospital, after reaching
the required five pounds.
The boys are two months old
in this photo. Scott is in
Ronnie's lap.

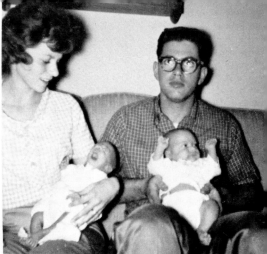

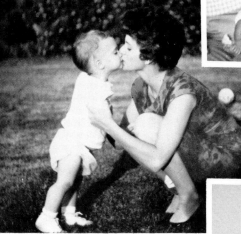

Scott, about one and a half
years old, giving me a kiss.

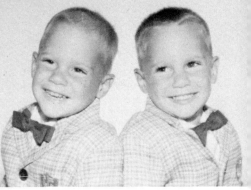

Steven and Scott at two years.

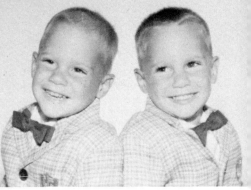

Scott and Steven posing on
the way to their first day of
kindergarten.

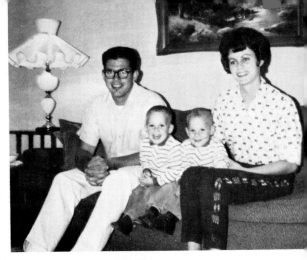

Ronnie, Scott, Steven, and myself in April 1963.

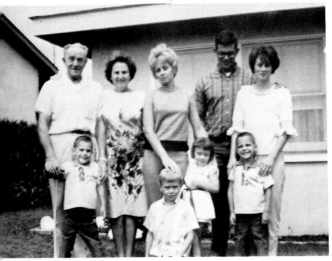

"Grandpa" Harry, "Grandma" Christine, Phyllis, Ronnie, myself, Steven, Mark, Kym, and Scott after a family barbecue.

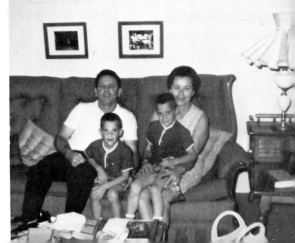

Ronnie's parents, Jack and Roma, with Steven and Scott.

Kym, Mark, Steven, and Scott
in a usual happy pose.

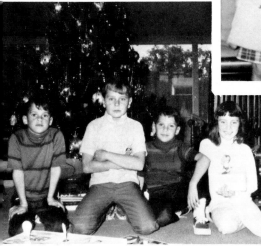

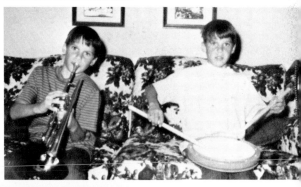

Steven, Mark,
Scott, and Kym at
their Grandma
Christine and
Grandpa Harry's
house on a
Christmas day.

Scott with his trumpet
and Steven with drum
pad a few days before
Scott's first hospitalization in October 1971.

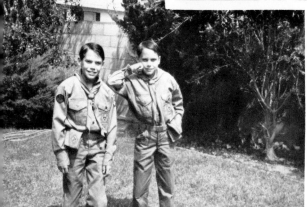

Steven and Scott in
June 1972 before a
Boy Scout meeting.

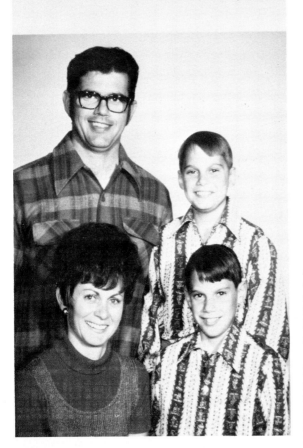

A family portrait
—Ronnie, Scott,
myself, and
Steven. Scott's
face is puffy from
medication.

Below: Leaning
against "Dad's
rotted piece of
junk" are Scott,
Mark, and Steven
ready to play
army.

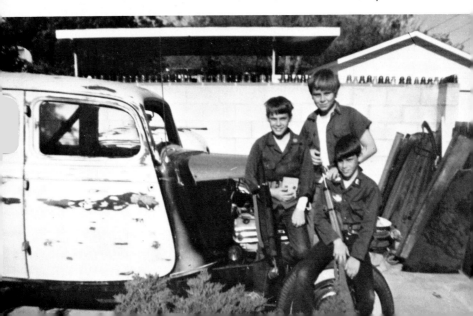

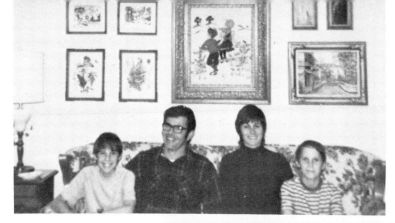

Thanksgiving 1974
at my mother's
house. Steven,
Ronnie, me, and
Scott.

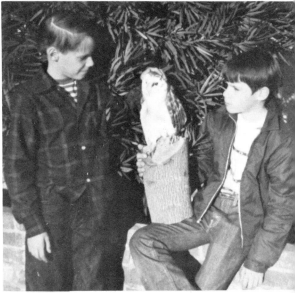

Scott, on the right, admiring
Steven's "stuffed" owl.

I took this photo of Scott by
the Sespe River, where we
stopped on the way to the
doctor's for his treatment.

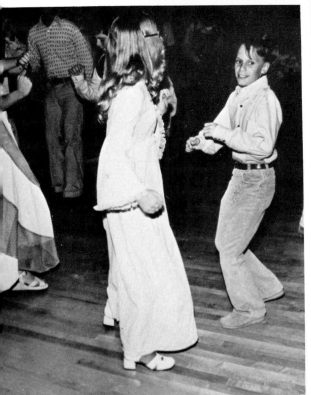

Scott proudly displays
his new fishing pole.

Julie Deeter dances
with Scott at a junior
high school dance.

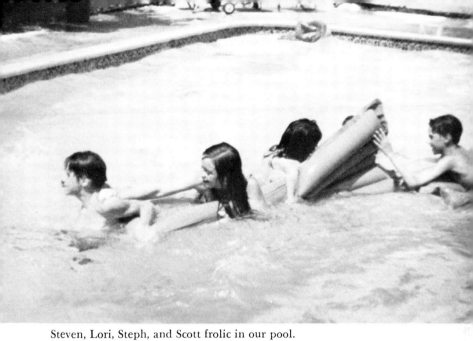

Steven, Lori, Steph, and Scott frolic in our pool.

Trampas unwillingly takes a ride in our pool, surrounded by Steven, myself, and Scott.

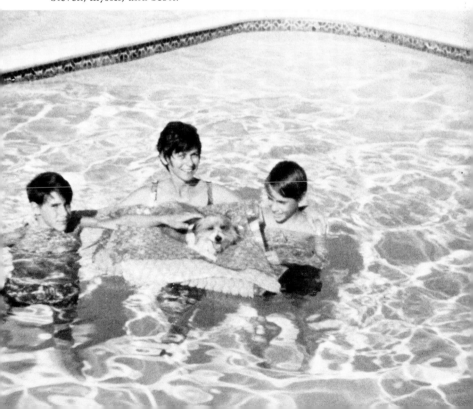

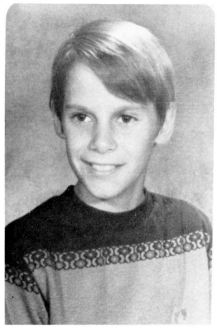

Scott's seventh grade class picture.

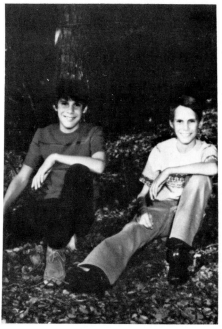

Photo of Steven and Scott during the eighth grade.

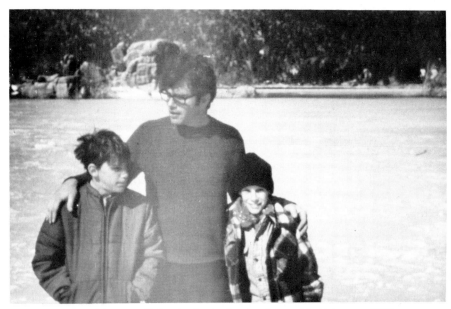

Frozen Big Bear Lake is the background for this February 1975 photo of Steven, Ronnie, and Scott.

Scott with his friends from Nuclear Medicine, "Woody" and Ken Day, in front of Children's Hospital.

Below: Jim and Jeff Fauver, Steven, Scott, and Webb McKelvy as they start out on their three-day Agua Blanca hike in May 1975.

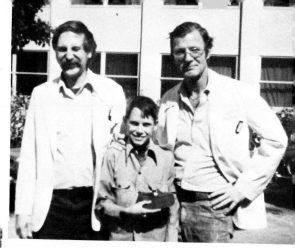

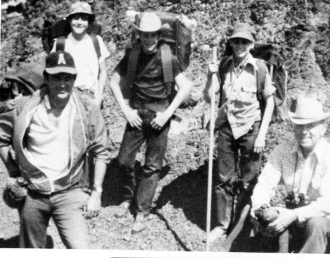

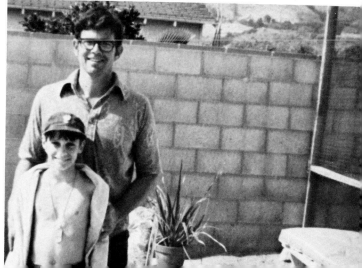

Scott and Ronnie after a swim by Scott in our backyard.

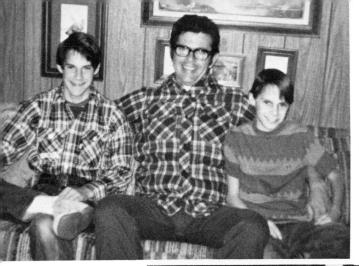

Steven, Ronnie, and Scott on Thanksgiving Day —our last with Scott—in November 1975 in our living room.

Myself, Steven, Scott, and Trampas, same day as above.

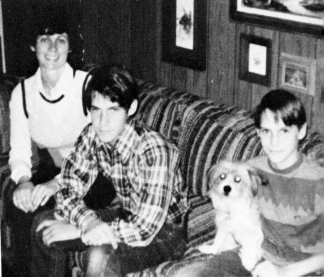

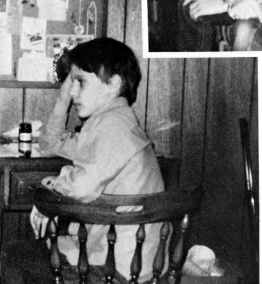

Scott at his desk.

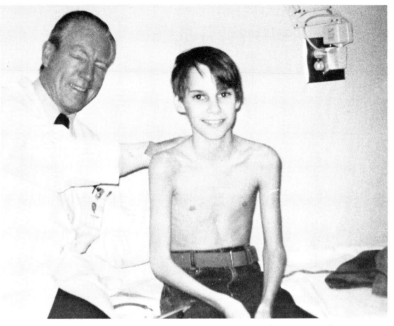

Dr. Kenneth Williams sitting alongside Scott during a February 1976 clinic visit.

This picture of Scott, taken by Steven in Yellowstone Park, August 1975, is Steven's favorite of his brother.

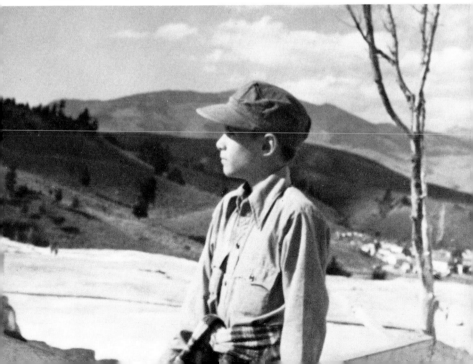

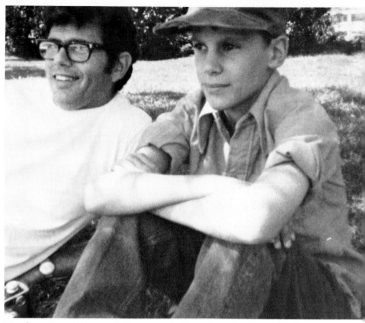

My favorite picture of Scott and Ronnie taken just a few months before Scott died.

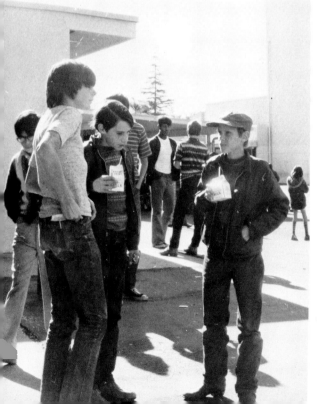

Outside the school cafeteria, Steven and Scott, then in the seventh grade, finish their milk while talking to classmate Eric.

Dr. Williams refers to this drawing as "Scott's shot tree." The army of syringes is carrying the Japanese flag and Scott is dressed in U.S. Army battle fatigues. Below the mountains, which overlook Fillmore, Scott drew Webb talking emphatically to his mules.

Scott's list of Important Days in the Hospital

IMPORTANT DAYS IN THE HOSPITAL

BY Scott

OCTOBER 29, 1971 ADMISSION TO GENRAL HOSPITAL, IN VENTURA.

NOVEMBER 4, 1971 NECK OPERATION PREFORMED.

NOVEMBER 8, 1971 ONE DAY RETURN HOME FROM VENTURA HOSPITAL.

NOVEMBER 9, 1971 ADMIDED TO LOS ANGELES CHILDRENS HOSPITAL.

NOVEMBER 15, 1971 OPERATION OF SPLENOCTOMY, LIVER BIOPSY, MULTIPLE LYMPH NODE EXTRACTIONS, APPENDOCTOMY PREFORMED.

NOVEMBER 10 or 11? 1971 LYMPH ANGIO-GRAM PREFORMED.

NOVEMBER 30, 1971 RELESED FROM LOS ANGELES HOSPITAL. HURRAH!

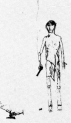

STICHES IN FEET 28
STICHES IN NECK 8
STICHES IN ABDOMEN 32
STICHES IN HIP 6

TOTAL STICHES 74

AVRAGE AMOUNT OF BLOOD DRAWS A DAY: 4
UNMESURABLE AMOUNT OF SHOTS A DAY
INJECTIONS: WEEKLY, DAILY, HOURLY, !?

TOTAL: UNCALCULATED!

OCTOBER 29, 1971 — ADMITTED TO GENERAL HOSPITAL OF VENTURA.
OCTOBER ? 1971 — BONE MARROW TEST PREFORMED ON STERNUM.
NOVEMBER 4, 1971 — NECK BIOPSY OPERATION PREFORMED.
NOVEMBER 8, 1971 — RELEASED FOR ONE DAY FROM GENERAL HOSPITAL.
NOVEMBER 9, 1971 — ADMITTED TO CHILDRENS HOSPITAL OF LOS ANGLES.
NOVEMBER 10 OR 11, 1971 — LYMPH ANGIO-GRAM OPERATION PREFORMED.
NOVEMBER 15, 1971 — SPLENOCTOMY, LIVER BIOPSY, MULITIPLLE LYMPH NODE BIOPSY AND APPENDOCTOMY
OPERATIONS PARFORMED.
NOVEMBER 30, 1971 — RELEASED FROM HOSPITAL. HURRAH!

NOVEMBER 24, 1971 — CHEMOTHARAPY. INJECTIONS, INJECTIONS, INJECTIONS! YUK!
JANUARY 22, 1973 — LAST INJECTION. HURRAH! YEA!

SEPTEMBER 9, 1973 — ADMITTED TO CHILDRENS HOSPITAL. AGAIN.
SEPTEMBER 10, 1973 — VERTABARA BIOPSY AND BONE MARROW OPERATION PREFORMED. AGAIN.
SEPTEMBER 11, 1973 — RELEASED FROM HOSPITAL. AGAIN.

OCTOBER 8, 1973 — ADMITTED TO CHILDRENS HOSPITAL. AGAIN. BLOOD TRANSFUSION PREFORMED.
OCTOBER 9, 1973 — NECK BIOPSY OPERATION PREFORMED. AGAIN.
OCTOBER 10, 1973 — RELEASED FROM HOSPITAL. FINAL!!!

OCTOBER 15, 1973 — NEW CHEMOTHARAPY TREATMENT STARTED. YUK!

STICHES IN FEET ———— 28
STICHES IN NECK ———— 8
STICHES IN ABDOMEN — 32
STICHES IN HIP ———— 6
                TOTAL   79
STICHES IN NECK AGAIN— 3
            NEW TOTAL 77

Scott's revised list up to October 15, 1973.

Scott apparently felt that he was being attacked by scalpels, syringes, I.V. setups, pills, and bandages when he drew this.

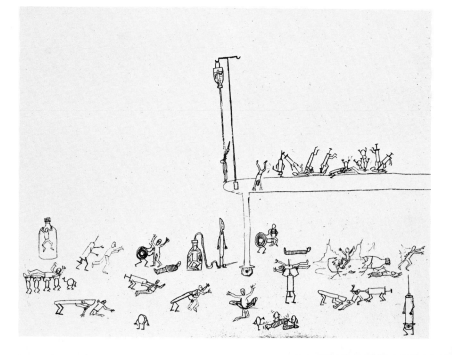

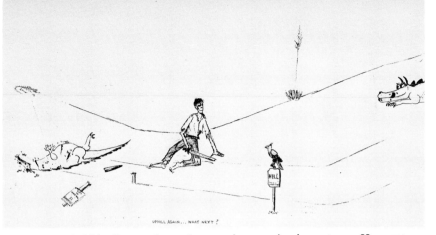

UPHILL AGAIN... WHAT NEXT ?

Scott battled his disease, shown here as dragons, in three stages. He went into a good remission and conquered his first dragon after treatment. He was barely over his second bout with the dragon Hodgkin's when he faced his battle with the third dragon. This battle proved to be fatal. In slaying the second dragon, he cut off the sign saying "Highway 13 . . . the road of life." The falcon, with a tear rolling from his eye, sits on a sign that reads "Hill (or Hell). This is a rough one!" Dr. Susan Bach, an authority on interpreting drawings by ill children, says that children often show the extent of their diseases and even predict when they are going to die through their drawings. I'm glad I didn't find this until after Scott died, although I was terribly upset to learn that he obviously knew what the future held for him.

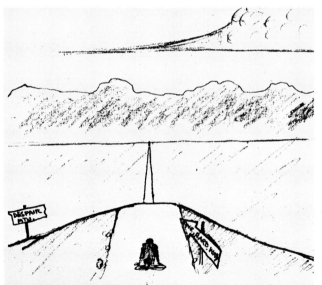

This small sketch was on the reverse side of his "Uphill Again" drawing.

THE LONG, HARD TRAIL... IT JUST WON'T STOP.

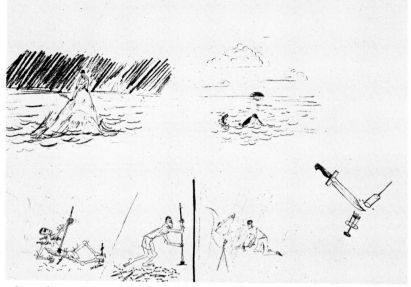

Scott sits atop a small island, his blue navy cap upon his head and stormy weather all around. The second frame shows just his cap left atop the island as the sun rises in a clearing blue sky.

The bottom of this page shows Scott with knives, needles, and a sword, which he pulls out to prepare for a battle with a robe-clad figure labeled "Death."

Scott may have been thinking of Dante's Inferno when drawing this.

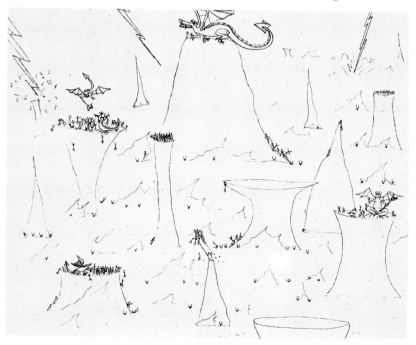

The trail was treacherously steep. We slid and tripped our way down. About an hour later, we reached a boulder-strewn side canyon with a few puddles of water. We dropped our packs and drank from the icy Agua Blanca. The water is the best I have ever tasted. We explored the area. We were amazed to see some fish dart around in the stream. We watched hawks. I found some chia and miner's lettuce.

We found a rake at the table, thoughtfully provided by the Forestry Service, and began to make ourselves some beds. They were amazingly soft. We spread our ponchos and sleeping bags over them. After we had beef stew for supper, went to the creek to wash up. I went down the trail alone and as I came back, Jeff growled from behind a rock and jumped out at me. I had been wondering how many wild critters there were in this canyon, so I let out a howl and took off.

Across the flat, there was a hill literally covered with blooming yucca plants. They looked like spirits of Indians drifting across the hills. We speculated on how terrified one might be if he heard voices coming from those ghosts. Just then some owls hooted. We drifted asleep in the moonshine.

The sun was rising on the hills above and on Cobblestone Mountain. White ashes swirled up from the fireplace. A large bird circled above the ridge, the sun striking its majestic wings. It was a condor. I hastily woke Scott and Jeff to show them the condor. We fixed breakfast—oatmeal, raisins and tea—washed up, packed up and hit the trail.

The further we went, the worse it got. Soon we got to Little Narrows. The place was shaded by the towering cliffs. They were gray cliffs and on one side there was a rock fall. We tried to go over the rock fall, but it was impossible. The other side of the wall went into the water at a steep angle. There were boulders in the creek, so we decided to go boulder hopping around the rock fall. After we crossed the creek, we took a look down the canyon. There were a thousand turns. Every turn we took, we thought would be the Narrows.

The trail was rougher and rougher with each turn in the creek. Scott and Jim hiked at about the same pace with Jim huffin' and puffin'. Even when we'd rest and I knew that Scott was tired, Scott would say to Jim, "Okay, let's go."

Soon we were going through dense brush and hopping logs in the creek. The canyon walls rose high above me. There were places where we could not walk through the creek bed due to small water falls, so we would go through the brush. Jim lost his fishing pole in the brush. After some hours, we arrived at the trail that went over the Narrows. That trail is about the steepest one I ever saw. So winding that one linear mile uphill was equal to about two miles of walking. The mountain was steep enough to make us be wary of falling off. The chaparral was thick on it and we saw many caves in the rocks.

The view that we got when we reached the top will stick in my mind to my dying day—an immense range of hellishly rough mountains as far as the eye could see. This was the kingdom of the chaparral.

On Sunday, they came home—tired, hungry, dirty, and happy. They had hiked twenty-five rough miles through Agua Blanca Canyon. "I don't know how Scott did it," Jim told us. "He kept up with us and never complained."

Chapter Eleven

Any hopes that were raised by Scott's ability to make the hike through Agua Blanca Canyon were dashed when he began having headaches and backaches again. His red blood count was low, too. We had to face the fact that he really was not getting any better. Scott himself realized that his Hodgkin's was not disappearing the way Duane Russell's had. Or Dr. Blodget's. And yet, we were convinced that Scott was getting the best medical care available. Why had God seen fit to cure Duane and Dr. Blodget and not Scott?

We finally decided to take Scott to a faith healer, something I had resisted earlier. It could do no harm, I thought now. It might do some good. There had been a lot of articles about people who had been cured by Kathryn Kuhlman, including children with cancer. As Ronnie said, "No one really understands about these healings. Let's ask Scott how he feels. If he wants to do it, we'll take him."

I was still sure that God could heal Scott anytime He wanted to, but I thought we should take him to Kathryn Kuhlman. If we didn't and if something happened (that's the phrase I always used to myself—"if something happened"), I would always think that if we had taken Scott to her, she might have healed him.

Scott was willing to go to one of her services, so the next thing was arranging to get in. You had to know someone in order to be assured of getting a seat. One of our friends said that I should take Scott in a wheelchair, because people in wheelchairs or on stretchers were admitted to a special section. But Scott did not need a wheelchair, and it did not seem right to cheat in order to get God's blessing. We managed to get an introduction and were told there would be seats for the four of us.

The atmosphere made me uneasy. I kept thinking that if she could really heal, how terrible it was for people to be turned away, people who, like us today, somehow thought God would listen to Kathryn Kuhlman, although He had not listened to them or to us. I kept looking over at the special section with people in wheelchairs and on stretchers. I was pretty sure I could recognize the children who had cancer. After you have seen hundreds of children with cancer, there is a look about them—quite apart from their hair loss and other external signs—that I used to call the cancer look. And I thought to myself— All right, if one of those children is healed today, I'll believe in faith healing.

At one point, Kathryn Kuhlman, who was up on a stage in front of us, said, "Someone here today is being healed of cancer right this very moment." My hopes quickened and I leaned over to Scott. "Are your nodes going down?" I asked. He was fingering them. "Not yet," he said.

There were persons there that day who believed that they were being healed. As each one of them came up onto the stage, the healer would say, "Remember it is not Kathryn Kuhlman who has healed you. It is the Holy Spirit." Many of those who claimed that they were healed testified that they had come unwillingly and had not been believers. One man said that he had fallen asleep during the service and when he awoke his varicose veins were healed. Another man claimed that he had been healed at Kathryn Kuhlman's services a month ago. He had had Hodgkin's and now his X rays proved he was free of the disease. I wondered if it was my skepticism that was keeping Scott from being healed.

We had thought the services would last for an hour, but they went on much longer. By the time they were over, both Scott and Steven were tired and anxious to go home. On the drive back to Fillmore, we discussed what we had seen and heard. I mentioned the way the healer kept saying that it was not she but the Holy Spirit who healed the ill and the crippled.

"Yes," said Scott, "but did you notice how she kept throwing her name in every chance she had?"

I decided that we had put Scott through a tiring day for nothing. We did not need a middleman between us and God. If He chose to heal Scott, it would be His will— and His answer to our prayers. But at least we had tried. And there were those who said that in some cases it took months after the healing services for the cure to be effected. I never stopped praying that God would heal Scott.

And my faith in Dr. Williams never wavered. He scheduled a series of tests for Scott "to see where we stand." Steven came along with us that day. Steven also felt at home in the hospital by now. A few months ago, he had had a swollen node in his groin and I had immediately been convinced that now he had Hodgkin's, too. But Dr. Williams had examined him and said he was fine. There was nothing to worry about. Since both boys were at the hospital, he asked if they would participate in a research project. "We're interested in learning more about the body's response to disease," he told them, "and whether or not having a disease or being on drugs the way you are, Scott, changes your immunity. We'd especially like to study you two, because you're identical twins."

We decided that if the study resulted in any discoveries that could help Scott or other children, it was important to participate. There were several tests, including a skin test that was slightly painful. Later on, Dr. Williams told us that Scott's white cells had reacted feebly and Steven's had reacted well.

I always encouraged Steven to come with us when it wasn't a school day. It was good for Scott to have company. And if Scott did not have a treatment, we would always do something "interesting" afterward. Usually we went to some of the little shops in Los Angeles that sold military items so Scott could add to his collection of medals and ribbons.

His favorite haunt was the store where Ronnie had found the miniature Purple Heart. The first time Scott went there, he told the clerk he was collecting battle ribbons and gave him the names of the ones he wanted to buy that day. The ribbons were in little drawers that had a picture of the ribbon in front. As the clerk started looking for the ones Scott wanted, Scott would say, "It's on your right" or "It's three drawers above." Finally the man said, "Why don't you just come behind the counter and pick out what you want?"

After that visit, they always let Scott go behind the counter. The owners told him that he could always count on a job at their store, because he knew their stock so well. They also carried camping paraphernalia and Steven would examine the various items he was interested in while Scott was looking at medals and ribbons.

But this day, the boys decided they wanted to go to the museum. Scott wanted to visit the radiation display and see if the isotopes from the bone scan he'd had that morning were still active. They were. We were about to move on to another display when a man walked up to the

Geiger counter. Scott walked past him and the counter started ticking rapidly.

The man, obviously surprised, held his watch up close to the counter. Scott walked away. The counter slowed down. The man started to walk away and Scott moved closer. The counter started ticking again. The man stopped and looked, then he shrugged his shoulders and started to leave. Scott moved closer to the Geiger counter and it ticked loudly again. The man turned. We were all smiling. He said, "I can't figure out what's making it go off." Scott told him and he laughed.

Then we went to look at a medal display. A few weeks ago when we had been there to see the same display, Scott had told me that he thought the Purple Heart that was shown was not correctly identified. Now he wanted to take another look.

Scott had read so much about medals that he had become quite an expert. One day he had taken his collection of medals and decorations to history class and given a talk about them. The teacher asked him to give the same talk to two other history classes.

The first thing I knew Scott was telling the guard that one of the medals was not correctly identified. The guard called the museum's military historian, Mr. Heerman, who came down to talk with Scott. Scott told him that he collected medals and thought that the one on display, which was described as a very rare purple cloth patch that George Washington had issued in August of 1782, was actually a medal that had not been issued until August of 1932.

Mr. Heerman thanked him, said he would correct the description, and invited him to look at the Honeywell collection of military medals and awards, which is not on public display. Scott was very excited when he spotted in the Honeywell collection one of the original Purple Hearts that was presented by Washington.

The *Ventura County Star—Free Press* ran a long story about this incident. In part, it said:

> Because of [Scott's] knowledge, the Los Angeles County Museum of Natural History now has been able to correct its description of an award on public display and has realized it is the owner of one of the rarest military awards on record. "I believe it is one of two," Scott Ipswitch said. "It is the opinion of historians that one such award was made in 1782 to a Sgt. Elijah Churchill and that it is in a private collection. The other two were presented to Sgt. William Brown of the Fifth and Sgt. Daniel Bissell of the Second Connecticut Regiment. One of those is in the Smithsonian Institution and the other one is in the Los Angeles Museum. I believe Mr. Heerman is finding out which it is." . . .
>
> Scott wrote about his feelings and experiences as a patient at Childrens Hospital and when the nurses, technicians and doctors in the blood disorder wards read it, they were most impressed. Scott's observations have now gone into print and they are required reading for new personnel, including interns who come to Childrens.

Most of Scott's writings are included here. He had started writing about his illness on his own when he was ten and eleven. Then in seventh grade, when he was twelve, his English teacher suggested he make up for work he had missed by writing about his hospital experiences. Scott had asked Dr. Williams some questions to make sure that his facts were right, and Dr. Williams had asked to see a copy of Scott's report when he finished it. One of the technicians, Ken Day in Nuclear Medicine, also read Scott's story and showed it to Mary Ames Anderson, who is head of public relations at Childrens.

Mary Anderson told me that Scott's story had so impressed everyone who read it that a hospital committee of administrators and doctors wanted to use it in their orientation program for interns. They felt it would help them understand what it was like to be ten years old and in the hospital.

Scott was overwhelmed when he got a letter from Drs. Plachte and Hansen of the Patient and Family Advocate Committee at the hospital. They wrote:

> Speaking personally for ourselves and for the other members of the Patient and Family Advocate Committee, we wish to thank you most sincerely for sharing your thoughts about your experience in this hospital. Your manuscript has given all of us, physicians, nurses, social workers, and other members of the hospital family, important information and insights which should enable us to help you and other patients in many aspects of effective medical care.
>
> All of us have been impressed with the honesty, clarity and poignancy with which you are able to express yourself in writing. Please do keep writing about yourself, your family, your friends and us. And do stay in touch with your friends at Childrens Hospital as we wish to get to know each other better, to share your joys as well as your anxieties, annoyances and frustrations. We would like to help you in every way possible, just as you can help us in learning better how to do our part.

Scott also showed his manuscript to Dr. Martin and Dr. Fletcher in Ventura. "It's very interesting," Dr. Fletcher told him. "I think it ought to be published. Maybe in a magazine. Certainly in a medical journal."

This impressed Scott a lot. And when we got home, he looked through the *Reader's Digest* and was further impressed by the amount of money that was paid for a "first person" story. "Mom," he said excitedly, "if I could get my story published, think of all the medals I could buy! I think I'll try."

"That would be nice," I said, thinking that it might not be nice at all. What if he really did get it published? I remembered Joanne telling me about the newspaper that referred to Richard as a "dying boy" when it ran an appeal for blood. I was afraid of an introduction by a magazine editor saying this was a story written by a dying boy or that Scott had cancer. No amount of money would be worth the heartbreak this might cause Scott.

I told him that since everyone who had read his story had suggested that he keep on writing, this was the thing to do. And when he was finished, I said I would type it for him. He did do more work on the manuscript, but after a few weeks, he seemed to forget about the idea of sending it to a magazine. I think he was more interested in writing about what was going on in the present and how he was feeling in the present than writing about the past.

One evening just before the end of school, Scott and one of his friends went to a potluck supper at our church. Colonel Heath Bottomly was the guest speaker. Scott was impressed by all the colonel's battle ribbons and decorations, and the colonel was impressed that Scott knew what they all were. Our minister asked Scott if he would be willing to introduce the colonel to the group before he gave his speech. So Scott did. Standing on a chair so he could point to each decoration on the colonel's uniform, he told the audience just what each one stood for.

"You really missed something," a friend told Ronnie and me the next morning. "You should have been there. There weren't many dry eyes in the audience. You know he received a standing ovation."

"Colonel Bottomly must have been pleased," I said.

"No, no. The ovation was for Scott!"

Chapter Twelve

Scott and Webb had become very special friends. They both understood what it meant to be in pain for long periods of time. Webb usually telephoned or came over the day after Scott had a treatment just to keep him from being too miserable. On sunny days when he knew Scott was not going to school because he was recovering from his treatment or had a cold, Webb would take him for rides to visit his friends on ranches and farms in the area. He made many days happy for Scott that otherwise might have been long and lonely.

He was always after him to "Get out in the sun. That'll help your punies, Scott." And he scolded him when he caught him eating candy bars. "Eat good food—oranges and apples. Not so many of these damn candy bars." And Scott listened to him. I'd come home from the store and find him sitting in the sun by the pool. He'd tell me, "Webb says it'll help make me strong and put color back in my cheeks."

Just a few days after the boys graduated from junior high school, Webb came by to propose what would turn out to be one of the greatest experiences Scott ever had. Webb told me that he was going to drive to Idaho to pick up his son Chris and he'd like to have Scott come along with him. He was going to visit a few friends on ranches and see some beautiful country. I told him that it sounded wonderful and I'd check with Ronnie and Dr. Williams and see what they had to say.

"It won't be hard on Scott," Webb said. "He can keep his sleeping bag unrolled in the back of my rig and rest whenever he wants. I travel different from most people. I don't make special plans with destinations I have to reach every night. If Scott gets tired, we'll stop. We may go three miles in a day or three hundred."

"When are you planning to leave?" I wanted to know.

"Tomorrow."

Tomorrow? That was Webb all over. Never mind. It would be a wonderful trip for a fourteen-year-old. I hated to say no. I was scared to say yes. I left it up to Ronnie.

"It sounds great! Of course he can go," said Ronnie.

"But he's just had his treatment. His blood count is low. What if he gets sick? What if . . ."

Ronnie interrupted. "What if he never gets a chance to take a trip like this again?"

Dr. Williams thought it was a great idea, too. So finally I asked Scott if he'd like to go. No question about it. He was all excited. And very proud that Webb had asked him to go along. He packed his duffel bag for the trip with the man that he sometimes called Ol' Fossil.

Ol' Fossil stands about six feet tall, kind of paunchy, a slight pot belly. He has a high forehead, receding grayish hair and a medium-sized nose. His eyes are hazel with high gray brows. His chin comes to a slight point. His bony cheeks stand out like an Indian's. His neck is wrapped with a bandanna.

The long-sleeved shirt he wears smells nicely of sage brush and is tucked into a pair of much-worn corduroy Levis. The western-style belt he wears has a homemade buckle bearing his snakelike brand. His ankle high boots are sometimes stained with mud. His sweat-stained straw cowboy hat is worn high on his head. A warm friendly smile gives a sense of welcome, his white, even teeth glistening with glints of gold.

When Scott and Ol' Fossil left, I gave Webb an envelope containing my parental consent for any medical aid Scott might need, a list of the medicines and doses Scott was taking, the pills he was to take, and his latest blood count, as well as a list of all the necessary phone numbers. They drove off with great smiles and waves. "He's going to be just fine," Ronnie said as he hugged me too hard after Webb's rig had turned the corner and disappeared from sight.

Scott kept a diary for the first three days of the trip.

June 18, 1975—Went through several towns that were just about ghost towns. Pretty sparsely populated. Went through Panamint Valley, saw several sidewinders, lizards and burros. Got pictures of burros. Hotter than hell in desert. Started coolin' off about 7:00 p.m. Camped at Wildrose Camp in Death Valley Monument. Seven short-eared owls flew right over us, just about gave us hair cuts. Seemed interested in our fire. Burros all over, braying to beat hell. Havin' some hot chocolate for dinner. Kinda tired, but feel fine. Beautiful half moon, clouds, dusk. Real neat desert country. Five flares seen over China Lake, floating down lighting whole place up.

June 19, 1975—6:00 a.m. Comin' out from Wildrose to Death Valley exactly six o'clock. We're 5,000 feet high and in a cold, cold desert. The sun's already up so it'll be gettin' warm soon enough. (7:55 a.m.) Ran out of gas. (7:57 a.m.) Blue car with old codger in it pulls up, gives Webb a ride to Furnace Creek. I see him go up over the horizon. (8:00 a.m.) Forestry Service car pulls up. I tell them the situation. They go off and disappear.

The wind is startin' to whistle, the sun is getting warmer. This must be the most desolate place around. I can just see the mule teams ridin' up the hill. The whole Death Valley is before me. Mountains to my right (west), towering peaks to my left (east). In front of me are more hills and mountains. Same behind me. This is desolate. I see nothing living all around me, save for a few dry grasses. Borax, salt, lethal, deadly. This is Dante's Inferno—Death Valley! Earlier this morning we saw lots of burros. There's an over-population of them. There must be literally hundreds of jackrabbits and cottontails within sight. One just about ran into me while I was brushing my teeth. He was a baby cottontail, wandered up to me, realized what I was and hurried off—not far, to a bush, and stayed there looking at me.

(8:15) Webb arrived back, gave the rig a gallon of gas and we're on our way. (8:20) Reached a gas station and we're filling the rig up. Boy, she's guzzlin' that gas. Soon as she's filled up, we'll go over to the cafe and get some long-waited for breakfast. Now I know why they call Furnace Creek, Furnace Creek. It's like a furnace here, and only 8:20 in the morning.

(12:20) Crossed the Nevada–California line. I'm in Nevada for the first time. (4:32) After touring Las Vegas and seeing some more vast desolate land and rocky barren mountains and dusty desolate hills, we are now in the State of Arizona. It's still dry and hot, but just saw first river with real water in it since leaving Kern County, California. (4:40) Am seeing beautiful work by highway engineers. Can see drill marks for dynamite which are perfectly straight and even. Not only did they move part of the mountain away, but they made it beautiful. Can see strata, etc. Makes you feel good that some-one in U.S. still not just wants to do the job and say, "Aw, just blast the hell out of it" but does the work artistically so that generations to come will still be able to witness and enjoy this beautiful canyon land. (5:10) UTAH! (7:00) In beautiful cedar country. Lava beds, mountains, hills, water everywhere. Everybody has guns in their trucks and cars, rifles and pistols and they are loaded. Not to shoot people or be ornery, but to be ready for deer, bear, etc. These are wonderful people. All Mormons. This would be a very, very nice place to live. Cattle country. Snow country. This, I think very seriously, is where I might want to live. The south western corner of Utah. Cedar City. Around there.

June 20, 1975—(1:20 p.m.) Hailstorm just outside Nephi, Utah. (3:00 p.m.) Salt Lake! There's a hailstorm going on so loud I can't hear myself think in this rig. The stones hittin' the window are about as big as my thumbnail. The lightning almost hit us! Well, it was about a mile off, but that's pretty damn close. The storm is over now, well, at least we drove out of it. There are actually some clear spots around the clouds. But I have a feeling that this storm ain't gonna leave Salt Lake City for at least a couple of days. (4:45) **IDAHO!**

There was no doubt but that Scott was influenced not only by Webb's appreciation of the natural world, but also by his way of expressing himself. Webb's destination was Coeur d'Alene, where his son Chris was staying with friends who had a place on the Saint Joe River.

Webb and Scott and Chris drove off to a ranch one day to look at horses. After Webb parked the rig, Scott decided he was too tired to hike into where the horses were pastured. He would stay with the rig.

"Okay," said Webb, "we'll be back soon. You know where the pistols are and how to use them. You never know what you might run across. There are a few weird people everywhere."

When Webb and Chris came back an hour or so later, they saw a man standing by Webb's rig talking to Scott. As they walked up, the man said, "You must be friends of his."

"Yeah," said Webb, "we are. Why?"

"I figured you had to be, because when I walked up, he pointed two pistols at me." Scott had been sleeping with the pistols by his side, and the man had startled him. The man, it turned out, used to live in Ventura County, so the four of them had a lot to talk about. Before the man left, he asked Webb, "Where did you get this kid?"

Scott would have been small for his age anyway. Steven was. But the drugs he took really stunted his growth. And this often surprised people who met "this little kid," and then heard him talk intelligently about so many things. Webb told me that wherever they went on this trip, his friends never paid much attention to Scott at first. But after a while, the men all accepted him as their equal. Webb said that a lot of his friends told him, "If you ever get tired of this kid, send him to me."

On the way back from Idaho, the three of them were thirsty after driving many hot miles through desolate country. They stopped at the first roadside place they came to. It was a café and bar. As they walked in, Scott noted a sign that said, "Children must stay in the booths." Webb and Chris went straight to the bar and ordered beers. Scott stood for a moment, looked at the bar, the booths, and the sign. It was ten o'clock in the morning. Then he went up to the waitress and said, "Do I have to sit in a booth?"

She smiled and said, "Young man, you can sit right up here with your friends. What will you have?"

"Milk," said Scott.

On Sunday, June 29, Webb's rig pulled up in front of our house. The travelers were home. Scott unloaded rocks and bones and feathers and porcupine quills, almost stuttering as he tried to tell us about everything at once. It had obviously been the trip of a lifetime.

One day not too long ago, Webb sat down to write about some of his friends and how they had lived and died with courage in the Pacific islands during World War Two.

I was writing about John who had had the Purple Heart pinned on him by Admiral Chester Nimitz in Hawaii, when I suddenly found myself thinking about Scott. And then I started writing about him.

And then there was Scott. He never made a beach head. He never laid there on the beach and watched the flag go up a coconut palm. Scott never saved anybody's life. I guess he never even did anything to make this country better or safer or richer.

But he sure made a lot of lives richer and better for those people who knew him. I don't send cards or thank-you notes. I don't even remember birthdays or anniversaries. But for many years on Memorial Day and the Fourth of July and the Eleventh of November, I generally stop a minute and think of a few good men. A few good men that very few people knew. Like only a few people knew Scott.

Some would think of Scott as a boy. But John was only a year older than Scott when that blockhouse buried him alive. Those men with guts had a chance and lost. Scott never had a chance and never got a medal.

Scott and I slept in the mountains high above Death Valley. We listened to the wild burros and watched the testing by the military over China Lake. We cooked our dinner and ate around a sage brush fire. We rode working horses at the Sparrow Ranch in Big Hole, Montana. We fished beaver ponds and loaded wild mules and trailered them all the way to California.

Scott fished the Saint Joe River in Idaho. We ate in logging camps and he-men saloons. Talked to wild hoss buckeroos on the Magdalina plains and slept in the back of the rig amongst saddles and tack and Scott never complained. I knew he was frightened at times. He was too smart not to be.

When we talked of the time in his life, when he would be a man, it was just understood that he'd be a naval officer. There was no doubt in his mind that he could cut the buck. He didn't talk of war or combat like most youngsters. He spoke of Command. Of the duties of a leader. He understood about valor and honor and guts. He had an uncanny feeling for the bravery of men under stress.

We stood in the lobby at El Toro Marine Base. Scott would "read" the campaign ribbons of every man and woman. There was no hesitation about rank, tours of duty, awards for gallantry, multiple awards or value of deeds to deserve the citations.

He told me with a grin how a passenger pigeon was awarded the Congressional Medal of Honor. How a soldier captured a single horse from a Nez Percé warrior and was awarded the nation's highest award for bravery. How Medals of Honor were presented twenty years after the battle—and of the many that were recalled for political reasons.

I have never known a person of Scott's age with the reasoning power and ability to understand courage. Even the men who fought in the great battles could not tell what courage was. They just had it when the time came. Scott lived courage every day.

I rank him with those "few good men," this kid who truly deserves a Medal of Honor.

Chapter Thirteen

Aʟʟ ᴛʜᴇsᴇ years, my greatest fear—apart from the overriding fear that Scott would not recover from Hodgkin's—was that somehow he would find out that Hodgkin's was cancer. I worried myself sick about the effect this would have on him and his will to fight the disease. My fear was as irrational as my fear that bears would attack him that day we had hiked toward the pine forest below San Cayetano.

One afternoon I walked into the living room where Scott was lying on the sofa watching television. There were slides of magnified cells on the screen.

"That's what I have," Scott said, without taking his eyes away from the television.

"What?"

"That's what I have. Cancer," Scott said.

"How long have you known that Hodgkin's was cancer?" I asked in amazement.

His answer was matter-of-fact. There was no hint of emotion. "Ever since I was in the hospital."

"Who told you?" I wanted to know.

"No one," he said. "I just figured it out from what the doctors said."

How I could have thought that Scott would not make

the connection between Hodgkin's and cancer is beyond me today. I knew what an inquiring mind he had. I knew that he had read everything in the public library about Hodgkin's. And that he had watched the children and listened to the conversations in the Hematology-Oncology Clinic for all this time. Yet, somehow I had believed that Scott did not know he had cancer. And I had believed that it was better for him not to know. I had fretted myself into uncounted sleepless nights and fits of crying worrying about what would happen if he found out—when he found out. How could I have so underestimated my son? In retrospect I suspect that our not telling him he had cancer was as much to protect ourselves as to protect him. But I don't know. I really don't know.

"Daddy and I didn't tell you what it was," I told Scott, "because we didn't want to scare you."

"I know," he said calmly. "I'm just lucky I have Hodgkin's." And turned his attention back to the television as the narrator described the different treatments for cancer—surgery, radiation, chemotherapy. At the end the narrator said, "Cancer will strike one family out of four this year."

Scott smiled at me. "Well, since I have cancer, that means there's one family that doesn't have to have it." I kissed him and he squirmed.

If only I had been the one stricken so the rest of my family could be spared. So often I had wished that it could have been me. I would have given anything to have taken Scott's illness on myself.

Scott seemed to want to cram every possible experience into that summer. After his big trip with Webb, he went off to our church camp at Hume Lake. The year before, he had been too ill and weak to go, but this year when I suggested that it might be wise for him to stay home because his hemoglobin count was dropping, he said,

"Heck, no, Mom. Nothing's going to keep me away this year."

Camp proved to be a meaningful religious experience for him. One of the pages in his notebook contained some thoughts on the death of Christ that he had written while at camp.

> **When nailed to the cross, the lungs would collapse and breathing was pure, terrible torture . . . Forty lashes with a cat-of-nine-tails would kill an ordinary man. They beat Jesus Christ 39 times. Literally within an inch of his life . . . Christ died of a broken heart.**

The next event was a family vacation trip to Yellowstone National Park. Scott planned our itinerary, poring over his maps and figuring out where we would camp each night. We planned to leave on a Saturday, the day after Scott had his treatment. He was not affected by them so much at this period and we felt he would be strong enough for the ride.

Scott was in high spirits when the doctor came into the examining room. "I'm in a big hurry," he said with a smile, "so let's get this over with."

"What's the big hurry?" the doctor asked.

"We're leaving on vacation tomorrow. We're going to go to Yellowstone and drive through Arizona, Utah, Idaho, Montana, Wyoming, and Oregon. We're going to camp and fish . . ." Scott broke off suddenly and asked, "Is my count okay? Can I have my treatment?"

My stomach began to tense. The doctor had seemed hesitant. Was he going to tell Scott he could not go?

"Well, your white count is good, but your red count is at the point where we wouldn't want to give you your treatment if it were any lower." He paused. "I'm going to give you your treatment, but since it's going to knock your low red blood count even lower and since you'll be traveling in high altitudes, I think you ought to get some red blood cells."

"You mean I have to have a transfusion?" Scott asked disappointedly. He had only had transfusions when he had surgery and sometimes there had been undesirable side effects. I asked the doctor to call Dr. Williams first to see if he thought it was a good idea.

Dr. Williams agreed, and the next day Scott was given two units of packed red blood cells. It was a long procedure. The first unit was dripped in very slowly over several hours to let Scott's body adjust to the new cells, then the second unit was administered a bit faster. After a couple of hours, Scott fell asleep and I sat watching his skin become tinged with pink. He looked beautiful. Truly beautiful.

The transfusion forced us to postpone our vacation one day, but it made Scott feel so much better that we all rejoiced. His added pleasure more than made up for the lost day. The trip through eight states was tiring, but Scott enjoyed every minute of it, and we decided we would have to return to Yellowstone and hike even deeper into the park.

On the way home, we stopped at Weed, which is near Mount Shasta, where the Russells lived. This was the high point of the vacation for me. Gladys Russell and I had corresponded for years, but this was the first time we had met. And when I met Duane, my heart was full of joy. He was strong and handsome and showed no signs of Hodgkin's. I told the Russells how much it had meant to all of us to know that Duane had had Stage Four Hodgkin's just like Scott and had been given the same drugs Scott had—and been healed. I hoped that our prayers would help heal Scott soon, just as Duane had been healed. And yet, I left with a sad heart. The contrast between Duane and Scott was cruel.

The boys' summer ended with a bang—or rather, a roar

of thunder. Steven described their "last fling." The day before school started, Steven wrote:

Scott, Jeff and I were determined to have some fun before we were enrolled in this somber institution. We planned a trip up Sespe Creek to go fishing.

Naturally the minute we got up at the crack of dawn, solemn clouds clogged the sky with damp tidings. I remember the old saying, "Red sky in the morning, sailor take warning." I glanced at the east. Blood red. Soon we headed up the road to the canyon. The red earth mingled with boulders strewn in the canyons and contrasted with the green of hillside vegetation. We walked up the creek talking about Mr. Westgate (our neighbor) and his warnings about staying out from under oaks during thunder storms. Heck, we were saying, it probably won't even rain.

As we walked farther, the trail got harder, the boulders grew bigger, the canyon got thinner and the sky grew darker. But by the time we got to Coldwater Canyon, we figured that it would never rain so we settled down to fish. We spotted big green turtles and good-sized trout. I got a bite and started to reel him in. As soon as I got him off the hook, big, fat, juicy raindrops splattered into the creek. They grew in size and intensity as we crawled under a nice, safe lightning rod, er, oak tree. Lightning struck.

We were out from under the tree as fast as I could say "Hell's Bells," which I did in a rather high-pitched voice. When we heard the thunder, it was low and rumbly, far up in the canyon. But as it came down, it bounced off the canyon walls and back down the canyon. The thunder shook us up a little, mainly because it was shaking the boulders out of the creek. But as soon as we got under a nice safe rock, the storm subsided and we found it pleasing to come out and fish again.

Time began to fly and we proceeded to fish our way down to the road. Just as we stepped into a clearing, we met two most interesting people. One guy was sprawled out on the sand, dreaming whatever his garbled mind could permit. The other stood in the middle of the stream with a jug of whisky in one hand and a pole in the other. Both wore nothing.

"Hey," said one of them, "y'wanna know what makes good bait?" Scott calmly showed his interest in what did make good bait. "Y'catch a little frog an' stick 'im on yer hook."

We took off home.

Jeff's mother and I had worried about the boys when it started to rain. I drove up the road half an hour early to the spot where I'd told them I'd meet them. They were walking down the road toward home, glad to see us. Scott told me just how scared they had been when the thunder echoed through the canyon— "I've never been so scared, not even when I was in the hospital."

And the next day, they went off to school. They were entering the ninth grade and Scott was entering his fifth year of Hodgkin's. The boy whom the doctors had said would probably die two years ago was not only alive, but intensely involved in life. He started his diary again.

> September 14, 1975—I am very happy and have high hopes for this next year. School, which started last week, is neat. I feel better than I ever have. I just know this is going to be a good year.
>
> September 15, 1975—My back was sore when I got up, but I went to school. Later that afternoon, I called Webb. Me & Steven went hunting with him with my 1851 Colt Navy .36 pistol.
>
> September 16, 1975—Steve, Jeff and I walked to the church on the corner, taking an instrument I had made out of two long wires from dad's welding kit taped together with the hook part of a clothes hanger. It resembled a wire sheepherder's hook. We sat down in the

bench, out on the sidewalk, trying to get enough nerve to ring the church bell with the hook. I went into the covered entrance porch. Jeff & Steve signaled all clear and I hooked the bell rope, then jerked as hard as I could. Just then the Reverend drove up and got out of his car. We split! We ran up the alley, across the field into Clay Street. The Reverend was still with us. Halfway to freedom, I stopped like a dummy and waited for the Reverend to catch up. He caught me, reprimanded me and left. Found Steve and Jeff hiding a block away. We spent the night at Jeff's and soaped and chalked seven cars that night.

September 19, 1975—Me, Steve and Jeff went to the police station to apply for the hunter safety course. Football game, Fillmore vs. L.A. Baptists. We won—36 to nothing. Live band dance after game.

September 21, 1975—A big antique car meet was taking place at Knott's Berry Farm, so Dad took Mom, Me, Steve and Jeff. After Mom bought us tickets and gave us our paychecks for working in the store, we went into Knott's and watched the can can dancers and roamed around "Western Village". We rode the stagecoach and, of course, a "bandit" stopped the stagecoach to rob it. We pulled our pocket knives on him. He shot at us. Steve & Jeff pretended to fall down dead. Two birds with one stone.

September 22, 1975—I'm starting to get a sore throat.

September 24, 1975—I woke up with a sore throat, so I didn't go to school.

Scott's temperature went up to 103 that evening. I called the Ventura Clinic and got the usual advice— "Two Tylenol and call if it gets worse." The next day I drove Scott over to Ventura to see Dr. Fletcher, who ordered a blood test.

Dr. Fletcher called me at home that night and said that Scott's hemoglobin was low and that his platelets had increased and were abnormal. He had called Dr. Williams about this and told me that Dr. Williams wanted me to bring Scott down to Los Angeles on Monday, September 29. "Scott's blood count is really undergoing some weird changes," Dr. Fletcher told me. "I think Dr. Williams will probably want to do a bone marrow. Don't mention it to Scott yet, but I want you to be prepared for it."

"What do you think is causing it?" I asked, scared to death.

"It could be due to his disease," he said. "Or he may have antibodies working against his red blood cells." My heart plunged. Please, God. Please don't let his disease take over.

Scott was feeling weak and still had a sore throat on Monday, when we went to Los Angeles. Dr. Williams examined him and said that his blood count was "really staying about the same." I could not understand this after what Dr. Fletcher had told me.

"His blood count hasn't really changed since the one in Ventura last week," Dr. Williams explained. "So I think we can hold off on the bone marrow for a bit. We'll run some blood tests to see if he has some antibodies that might be causing the low red blood count. It could be that. Sometimes Hodgkin's patients develop antibodies against their own red blood cells. You bring Scott back in two weeks and we'll start some new blood tests."

Scott began to have backaches again, just like the ones he'd had a couple of years before. Back rubs and Tylenol helped. Ronnie thought that his back probably hurt because he'd been lying down so much lately. But I was worried. I couldn't sleep. My stomach was always upset. And I couldn't even think of eating. Most nights when Ronnie and I made love, I would burst into tears afterward. I kept thinking that Scott would never grow up to know the joys of lovemaking.

When we went back to Childrens, Scott's blood count

was a little better and his red blood cells looked more normal. But the backaches continued. The next time we went to Childrens, one of the hematologists noticed some pus in Scott's throat and did a culture. It might be that it was an infection that was driving down his red blood count. They also scheduled more X rays, a bone scan, and one of those hated bone-marrow tests.

> **Was injected with isotopes for my bone scan, then went to get my marrow sucked out. They used a dull needle. The nurse had to apply every bit of her most plentiful weight just to get the needle through my skin. It took almost five minutes for her to work it into my bone. Finally she got it through. Up to now it didn't hurt too much. I had moaned a little, but it wasn't too bad. Then they stuck a needle in to get a bit of bone for the biopsy. It was awful, but I held back my screams as well as I could, moaning a little.**
>
> **But that wasn't the worst of it. She put in another needle through the main one to get the marrow. The pain defies description. I screamed a blood-curdling shriek. It left me exhausted, motionless. Then they had to take another syringe full, so I steeled myself for it. Again, terrible excruciating pain. I screamed and when it was over in about thirty seconds, I collapsed from my rigid position into a motionless blob. I was heaving to breathe.**

I had stood at Scott's head during the bone-marrow procedure, holding his arms while one of the hematology nurses held his legs. It was almost unbearable watching that nurse try to thrust the dull needle—these are the quarter-inch hollow needles—into his skin and through the bone.

After it was all over, the nurse had Scott feel the needle. She showed us how dull it was and apologized, saying that she could not touch it beforehand to test it for sharpness or it would not be sterile. The next time I saw her, she said that she had sent all the needles out for sharpening. I felt that there must be better ways of determining whether or not needles are sharp than by torturing a patient.

Scott had not received any treatments since the beginning of school. The doctors had decided not to start them again until they found out what was keeping his blood count down. Later that month, when Scott went to Childrens for his blood test, they were not able to get enough blood. The technician tried several times on each arm and was able to get only about five cc's—and they needed twenty cc's. When we left the lab, Scott had bandages on both arms and was trying hard not to cry.

Suddenly he exclaimed, "Mom! Oh, no! Look at my arm!"

There were two lumps, each the size of an egg, on his left arm. We rushed back to the lab.

"Oh, my gosh," the technician said, "get a hematologist to look at it immediately." So we rushed over to the hematology clinic, showed his arm to a nurse, and told her that Scott needed to see a hematologist as soon as possible. She nodded and stayed just where she was while we sat down to wait.

Scott watched her. In a few seconds, he said, "Mom, she hasn't called a doctor. Will you please tell her to hurry?"

"Honey, we asked her. I'm sure she'll get one in a minute."

Minutes passed. Scott said, "Mom, it hurts so bad. Please tell her to get a doctor quick." I was still hesitant. I didn't want to nag. I had made it clear that this was an emergency and she could see that Scott was in pain. But she had not made a move to call a doctor, so I went over and told her that Scott was very upset and that his arm was very painful.

"Dr. Morris will be back from lunch in a little while," she said. "As soon as he gets here, I'll tell him," she finished sharply.

We waited some more. The hematology nurse who had done Scott's bone marrow with the dull needle a few days before walked by and asked Scott what was wrong. He showed her his arm.

"I want a doctor to look at it," he said, "but no one will call one for me." The nurse didn't say anything, but she went away for a few seconds and came back with a cold compress that she held against his arm. Finally Dr. Morris arrived. He looked at Scott's arm. "All you can do," Dr. Morris told Scott, "is keep a cold compress on it and keep moving it. It's going to hurt when you exercise it, but you have to."

The next day Dr. Williams called me in Fillmore. He had good news. The bone marrow showed no sign of Hodgkin's. And he had bad news. The bone scan showed an area in the lower lumbar region that was brighter than the rest. It was exactly where Scott's back hurt. He wanted Scott back at Childrens in three days for more blood tests.

All this time Scott was trying to keep up with his schoolwork and doing well in spite of all the days he had to miss. He was chosen freshman senator to the Student Council. The Student Council adviser, who had previously worked as an aide to the late Senator Charles Teague in Washington, came to talk with Ronnie and me one evening. He thought Scott would enjoy going to Washington to serve as a Senate page and told us that he was sure it could be arranged. "Scott is just the kind of youngster who will get a lot out of the experience," he said.

Ronnie and I decided not to tell Scott right off, but

wait and see what happened. We didn't want him to get excited and then be disappointed. But I did ask Dr. Williams about it, and he assured me, "There's no problem. We can arrange for Scott to have his treatments in Washington." This buoyed me up. Even though Scott was feeling bad, even though they had discovered that suspicious spot in his lower back, we were talking seriously about something that Scott would be doing next spring. It was like a guarantee that Scott would be with us in the spring.

Just before Thanksgiving, Dr. Williams said that the blood tests had turned up two antibodies in Scott's blood. It might be that they came from the transfusion he had received in August before we went on our vacation, so he scheduled more tests to check it out. One of the hematologists who was present when Dr. Williams told us this said, "Scott, did you ever think you're anemic because of all the blood we take from you?"

"Yes," he replied, "I think you ought to let my blood alone."

His shoulder began to hurt, then his chest. And the day after Thanksgiving Scott was running a fever—so high that I rushed him to Ventura where the doctor said he had "some pneumonia." This meant more blood tests to find out what kind of pneumonia. When we went to Los Angeles, Dr. Williams said that Scott might have "walking" pneumonia. "You know, Scott," he said, "in World War Two, we used to see a lot of men just out of combat who had been fighting while they were suffering from this kind of pneumonia. We used to call it 'soldier's pneumonia' back then." He smiled at Scott and said, "If anyone would get soldier's pneumonia, it would be you." And Scott smiled back.

A couple of days later, I had to take Scott to Dr. Martin in Ventura again, because he was coughing so hard. Dr.

Martin checked him, told him to drink lots of juice and to cough as much as he could to keep his lungs clear. Just a few hours after we got back home, Scott started coughing and choking and asked me to call Dr. Martin again.

"But, Scott," I protested, "he said that you needed to cough."

"Mom, I'm afraid I'm going to choke," Scott cried. "I'm afraid I might die!"

He had never said anything like this before. Not in all those long years. I ran for the telephone. Dr. Martin said to bring Scott to the hospital immediately. When we got there, Dr. Martin ordered some antibiotics and said he was to spend the night under a mist tent. The nurse came in with a medicine tray and gave Scott a pill.

"What's this for?" he asked.

"It's the medicine Dr. Martin ordered for you," she said.

"I know. But what is it for?" he persisted.

"Scott, just take it," I said impatiently.

He shook his head worriedly. "Not until I know what I'm taking, Mom. They might give me the wrong stuff."

I thought of all the times that Scott had been right. He knew more about hospital errors than he should have had to know. I remembered the time the doctor had taped his IV in wrong. And the time his IV had almost run out because no one had checked it. If it hadn't been caught just in time, they would have had to start a new IV in a new vein. And I thought of all the times the technicians had butchered his veins because they had not paid attention to what he had told them about taking his blood.

"He has a right to know what he's getting," I told the nurse. She was exasperated, but she told him what each pill and liquid was for as she gave them to him.

I could not blame Scott for being frightened and rebellious. He had good reason.

Chapter Fourteen

I was frightened and rebellious, too. I also had good reason. Early in November, I had felt a lump in my breast. I was not only frightened, I was angry. I had no time for cancer. I had to be well for Scott. Now more than ever, since Dr. Williams had told me that they would be doing a biopsy after Christmas to see if Scott's Hodgkin's was active. I had to be with Scott when he had the surgery.

I knew that if that lump was not benign and I had to have a mastectomy, it would take time to recover. My doctor had been reassuring, saying that he would be surprised if it turned out to be malignant. But I was so certain that it was malignant, I would have been surprised if it had been benign.

Now here was Scott in the hospital under a mist tent. And I was scheduled to come to the hospital the next day for my biopsy. A few hours after Scott was discharged from the hospital, I was admitted.

As I was wheeled into the operating room, I remembered Scott's descriptions of how he had felt in similar situations. I refused to let myself be afraid. I had to be as brave as my son. Or try to be. I woke up with several nurses pulling and tugging at me. I tried to move, but someone said, "Just lie still." Then I saw my surgeon's face. In a voice that seemed to come from a faraway place, he said, "It was malignant. I had to do a modified radical." I was not even sure that he was talking to me. I closed my eyes. Later, I opened them and asked a nurse, "Did he say it was malignant?"

"Yes, he did," she answered softly.

Malignant. Well, there was nothing I could do about it. The next time I opened my eyes I was back in my room. My sister was there and Ronnie and my mother. I was so groggy I could not speak, but just lay there with my eyes closed. I was aware of everything they were saying.

"Do you think she knows yet?" my sister was asking.

"I don't know," Ronnie told her. "The doctor told her, but I don't know how conscious she was." I wanted to tell them that I knew and it was all right. I remember feeling terribly sorry for Ronnie, and wondering if God was answering my prayer of "Let it be me, not Scott." And if He were, was I really ready to die? My thoughts were racing, although I was too tired to talk. I wanted to live. But if God had decided to take me and let Scott live, I could accept that. It was very frightening to think that what I had prayed for might actually be happening. But would God save Scott? He would not take both of us, would He?

By evening, I was stronger and could talk. The surgeon came in and told me it would be a few days before they knew whether the cancer had spread. I was just as sure that it had not spread as I had been sure that the lump was malignant in the first place.

In a few days, I was well enough for Scott and Steven to visit me. I told them that the doctor had said I might have to have radiation or chemotherapy if they discovered it had spread.

"I know how you'll feel if you have to have chemotherapy," Scott said. "I can help you after your treatments when you're feeling sick. Just the way you helped me," he said earnestly. Then he smiled. "They're not too bad, Mom."

The next day the doctor came in with a big smile. "Your biopsies were all negative," he said. I had known that this was the way it would be. It looked as if I would have to spend Christmas in the hospital. Scott wrote me a letter saying, "If you can't come home for Christmas, we will give you some presents and have a small Christmas at the hospital for you. And we will keep the tree up and have Christmas when you come home, too. I'm thinking of you and I know how you feel in a way. I hope you aren't hurting too much. I know you'll get better soon. Don't worry about me. Just concentrate on getting well. I'm doing fine. I love you and hope to see you soon."

And Steven wrote, "I miss you and hope you'll be feeling better. I'm glad I got to visit you. Since you've been gone, the house got messy and the clothes and dishes were unwashed. So as usual I'm reminded how important you are around here. We got everything straightened up today. I hope you'll be out by Christmas. If not, I'll bring all your presents to the hospital."

Ronnie and Scott came to the hospital Christmas Eve and brought a few presents for me to open. Scott was cheerful and kept assuring me that I would feel much better as soon as I got home. He told me that he was feeling really good. But months later, I found a small scrap of paper in Scott's room dated December 24, 1975.

I'm tired. I hurt. I have double pneumonia, bronchitis, mononucleosis, two elusive antibodies, a head cold. My Mom is in the hospital and I just got out of the hospital. If things keep up like this, I just might get discouraged.

The doctor came by very early Christmas morning. "How would you like to go home today?" he asked. I beamed. "It's my Christmas present to you," he said with a smile. The boys and Ronnie picked me up at the hospital and we went straight to my parents' house for an early Christmas dinner. We all opened presents and exclaimed over them. It was a real Christmas. But by the time I got home I was on the verge of tears, and once safely in my own bed and the door closed, I gave way and cried. I was crying for myself. I was crying for Scott who looked so pale and was so tired. I was crying for people everywhere who were dying from cancer. For children who had not received any presents this Christmas. For my own physical pain. I was crying for Steven.

When Ronnie and Scott had come to the hospital Christmas Eve, I had asked where Steven was. They told me he had gone to the candlelight service with Webb McKelvey's family. The next day I asked Steven if he had enjoyed the candlelight service. "Yes," he said, "I liked it a lot. But afterwards when the McKelveys brought me home, I asked them in for some tea. I think they thought I was just trying to be polite. But I really did want company. I didn't want to be alone on Christmas Eve. I was glad when Dad and Scott got back."

Now I thought again about how often Steven must be and have been lonely with so much of my attention focused on Scott and with Scott's energies concentrated on battling his disease.

And I was crying for Ronnie. Ronnie who had to be strong for all of us and conceal his own pain while he pretended that everything was going to be all right. I had told Ronnie how sorry I was for him because I had lost a breast. "Don't worry," he said, "all I want is you and for you to be well." And I was sure he meant it. But it could not have been easy for him. And later on, he told me, "I wondered how many more things would happen to us."

I just had to get all those tears out of me. Ronnie came in and held me. He had learned over the years that I needed the release of tears. Many nights, once we were in bed, I could not hold them back any longer, and Ronnie would put his arm around me and cuddle me as if I were a baby. "There, there," he'd say. "Don't cry so hard. You'll make yourself sick."

And I had. I had made myself sick. I had been sick for more than four years now. All the time that Scott had been sick. Even in the earliest days, I would wake up before dawn and have to rush to the bathroom with nausea and diarrhea. And even though I took tranquilizers, I had never completely gotten over this early-morning sickness. A pattern had been established. Cry at night. Vomit in the morning. And live through the day on nerve and determination.

I have read that some doctors believe cancer is the body's response to intolerable emotional strain. In my case, perhaps it was. I was worn down to such a thin edge that it was a wonder I had not succumbed to any serious illness during these years. I had had a whole series of bad colds and sore throats, but nothing that had prevented me from taking care of my family.

After this night's outburst of tears, I felt calmer, and I recovered from my surgery very fast. Except for the one bad moment when Ronnie saw my wound for the first time, the loss of my breast honestly has never bothered me. I think— Well, this is what happened and I'm lucky. It could have been much worse. I don't feel sorry for myself. One of my friends who counsels women who have had breast surgery came to see me and we spent all afternoon talking. As she was going out the door, she stopped and said, "Oh, I didn't ask you how you were feeling. I keep forgetting you have had breast surgery." And I said, "Well, I forget that I have had it, too. I remember in the morning when I put my bra on and at night when I take it off. But that's it. Sometimes I will scratch my breast and Ronnie will say, 'Wrong one, honey.' "

I'd like to assure other women that I really do not think about it and that it has made no difference. Not in my life. Not in our marriage. I am blessed that I have such a loving and understanding husband.

What did bother me dreadfully was losing the use of that arm at first. The hospital therapist had given me a set of exercises to restore muscle function and strength. And I hated them. They hurt. One of the worst exercises involved creeping my fingers up the wall, trying to raise my arm a fraction of an inch higher each time. I got terribly discouraged. I was sure I'd never be able to raise that arm as far as my shoulder, let alone above my head. I can now. There's very little difference between my "good" arm and my "bad" arm.

And I owe it to Scott. He was a terrible pest and prodded me to do the exercises. When I wanted to stop, he'd say, "Come on, keep on, Mom. You can reach a little higher." And when I was working in the kitchen and I'd reach for something with my good arm, he'd say, "Mom, use your other arm. It will strengthen it." I used to get terribly exasperated with him. But he was right. And how could I refuse to try to raise my arm just a little higher or do a hated exercise just once more after all the painful tests and surgery and treatments that I had told Scott he had to have?

Chapter Fifteen

Early in January, Dr. Williams asked Dr. Woolley, the surgeon who had performed Scott's staging operation, to look at Scott's nodes and decide which node should be removed and when. After his examination, they decided that the biopsy did not have to be done immediately. "In a few weeks," said Dr. Woolley. "Perhaps a month or two," said Dr. Williams. Either way it was a reprieve.

Dr. Williams asked Scott if he had been doing any more writing, and Scott said that he had done very little since the beginning of his freshman year in high school. "I've been meaning to do some," he said, "but I just haven't."

"If you do, I'd really like to see it," the doctor said. "Will you show it to me?"

"Sure," Scott said. "I'll write some stuff up for you." And Scott began to spend more time writing. He had a green notebook in which he wrote "things for Dr. Williams." If I came into his room while he was writing, he would cover it with his arms.

"What do you want?" he would ask, annoyed.

"I was just checking to see if you were awake," I'd say.

"Well, I am," Scott would answer shortly and wait for me to leave the room. He spent most of his afternoons in his room now, reading and writing and listening to music. He'd often be asleep when I looked in on him. I'd tiptoe over and put a blanket over him. I had learned never to turn off his record player. A couple of times when I thought he was asleep, I'd turn it off. Without opening his eyes, he'd say in a monotone, "Leave it on. It helps me sleep."

It was months before I read what he had written in his green notebook. And when I did, I was very moved. It was much different from the little essays and reports he wrote for school. Much more revealing and much, much more mature. It was only natural. Scott felt more comfortable with adults than with his schoolmates. His illness had aged him far beyond his years.

An imaginary book report that Scott wrote for his freshman English class was representative of the writing he turned out for school.

Title: *The Sespian*
Author: *Scott Ipswitch*
Plot: *The life story of an interesting character*
It starts out when he was about 9, the time he moved to Fillmore. Before that his life, so much as he can remember, was relatively dull. Since the first grade he liked to read, especially about dinosaurs and war. He was a staunch introvert and unsociable.

When he moved to Fillmore, he was still introverted and moving did not help much. But he liked Fillmore. It was a small town. His grandparents owned a shoe store there and there were neat hills and mountains to explore.

Then in the fall of 1971, he began to get something. After a few months in the hospital and enough surgery to butcher several cows, it was discovered that he had a

slight disorder of the lymph system, namely Hodgkin's
disease. So he was treated for it and after a long struggle,
which is another book in itself, he was cured. He had a
wonderful summer that year and went hiking, camping
and other neat stuff. But, alas, it didn't last long. By
winter he was undergoing more surgery and tests. He
was having a relapse.

He was put back on treatment, a harsher medicine
this time, but he could not take the medicine and stay
alive at the same time, so they took him off this medicine. He did better, but was still getting sick and catch-
ing pneumonia. So the doctors put him on a better
treatment program. Slowly he got better and better. He
was hiking and in school and all—even when getting
treatments. This obviously was the treatment course for
him.

Since now he was able to spend at least half his life
normally, going to school, hiking, etc., he became more
un-introverted. In fact, he even started to like people.

Presently he is off of his treatment due to an unknown
anemia and is having lots of tests done in the hospital.
Besides the physical anguish of this ordeal, he also
undergoes mental anguish. His mood changes from depressed to happy to confused. He is probably in a few
ways crazy.

Scott's teacher gave him a good mark for this imaginary
book report, but I wonder what he would have thought if
he could have read Scott's entries in his green notebook.

January 8, 1976—While Danse Macabre is resounding
in my ears, I watch a pitiful sparrow on the front lawn.
The sky is a crisp, pure blue. The bare trees, with but a
few dead leaves. The mountains quietly sunning themselves. Such a magnificent day. Yet I languish in mental
and physical agony and torment.

I listen to Danse Macabre, the New World Symphony,
Prokofiev's Fifth. And I interpret them all as languish-

ing and agony. Why? Could it be because I have been anemic and in pain and in a progressively worsening condition for four months? Undergoing futile tests to try and determine the cause? Because I have two unidentified antibodies in my blood? And have had pneumonia for about three or four months? Because my lymph nodes are swelling and I face a possible lymph node biopsy?

Yes, this is why. Who can blame me for my recent short temper and moodiness? How I long to be free from this. Last summer was so wonderful. Why did it have to end like this? Nobody understands me.

If I were not used to such torment and pain, if I were like any normal person, I could have gone crazy long ago. Tearing out my hair. Screaming. Weeping pitifully. Yet, maybe I am. Maybe I am crazy. Yes, I am. Why is it so?

Just five days later, Scott and Steven celebrated their fifteenth birthdays. It was almost miraculous. It was four years and two months since Scott's Hodgkin's had been diagnosed. Two years and two months more than the life span the doctors had predicted. I prayed that we would see our boys celebrate their sixteenth birthdays together. I asked Scott what his birthday wish was.

"I think you know," he said, his brown eyes looking deep into mine.

"I'm sure I do," I said, hugging him. "It's my wish, too."

His backaches were getting worse. Dr. Williams prescribed a stronger pain pill and he was able to keep going to school until the end of January. Then he started running a temperature. There was no part of Scott's body that did not hurt. His head ached. His throat was sore. His shoulder hurt. His chest hurt.

At the end of January I took Scott to Ventura. His red blood count was way down, and Scott himself said that he felt miserable. While the doctor was checking the blood tests and X rays, he told Scott that if he didn't feel better soon, a stay in the hospital and a little oxygen might help. Then he had to leave the room to take a telephone call.

"Mom," Scott said weakly when we were alone, "if oxygen will make me feel better, will you tell him to put me in the hospital?"

"You're sure you want to go?"

"Yes," he said sadly.

And that afternoon Scott was back in the same room he had shared with Monty so long ago during his first hospital experience more than four years ago when no one knew what was wrong with him. He was very sick now. Afternoons, his temperature was 103 and 104. They gave him a blood transfusion and started an IV dripping antibiotics and vitamins into his system.

He was in the hospital for a week. When Dr. Martin told me that he could go home, he added some ominous words: "Scott seems to have bounced back," he said. "He's been able to bounce back from these bouts so often. It's really remarkable. But we have to understand that he might not always be able to. We shouldn't get to where we always expect it."

"What are you trying to tell me, Dr. Martin?" I asked. I knew what he was saying, but I didn't want to know.

"I'm not trying to tell you anything," he said. "Scott may never get pneumonia again. But if he does, well, we'll just have to deal with it when it comes."

Scott had an appointment with Dr. Williams the day before Valentine's Day. He was feeling pretty good. Just a couple of days earlier, he had come into the kitchen all excited to show me that his nodes were smaller. "Maybe I won't have to have the biopsy," he said as we were driving to Los Angeles.

After Dr. Williams examined him, he said Scott would

have to have the biopsy, but it could wait until after the first of March. He told Scott that they would also do a bone-marrow test and a bone biopsy, as well as the lymph node biopsy. Scott listened quietly. When Dr. Williams finished telling him about the surgery, Scott looked more depressed than I had ever seen him.

"What's the matter, Scott?" Dr. Williams asked gently.

"I don't want to have another operation." Tears rolled down his face.

Dr. Williams put his hand on Scott's leg. "It's the only way we can be certain whether or not your Hodgkin's is active," he said. "You know that."

"I know, but it'll just make me weaker."

Scott was silent, struggling for control. After a minute or two, his voice level, he asked, "Dr. Williams, do you know of any exercises I could do to build myself up?"

It was all I could do not to cry. There was nothing to build up. Scott was fifteen, but he was so short and so thin that people took him for nine or ten until they looked at his face. It was ageless. Drawn, strained, but somehow beautiful. Not an old face, but a face that reflected pain and control of pain. And his eyes were wise and understanding, not the eyes of a fifteen-year-old.

Dr. Williams answered him very seriously: "No, I can't give you any exercises at this time, Scott. But, if your nodes are enlarging because of Hodgkin's, Velban might be of some use. It's a less toxic drug than vincristine. Patients usually gain weight on it. If you gain weight, we can start talking about some exercises for you."

Scott brightened. So did I. Even this slim hope was something to cling to.

If I had been able to read Scott's green notebook earlier, I wonder if I could have helped him. I honestly did not know how to act and how to talk to Scott about his illness, even after I learned that he knew he had cancer. Hè did not seem to want to talk about it. And I observed his wishes, although I wondered if he was afraid and if I should talk to him about his fears. But what could I have said? That I was afraid, too? I could not have told him not to worry, that everything would be all right. What I did do was tell him that whenever he wanted to talk to me about anything at all, I was always there to listen. But he never talked about this one subject that filled my heart. And, as I learned from his writings, filled his, too.

A psychologist at Childrens Hospital asked me once if I could handle it if Scott asked me if he was going to die. I lied. I said yes. I read everything I could find about death and dying, hoping I would find answers to give Scott if he ever asked the question.

But he never talked about death. He loved to go shooting and he was an excellent marksman, but he never seemed able to hit rabbits when he went shooting with Webb and Steven. He shot one once and it upset him so that he never shot another. And he asked me to make Steven stop shooting birds in the backyard with his BB gun. But these were the only indications I had that death was more unsettling to him than it might be to another adolescent boy. When I read a paper that he left on top of his desk one day, however, I discovered that he had been keeping many feelings and thoughts to himself.

At first I was pale and I grimaced in pain. I was not as accustomed to pain then as I am now. I showed it and other people showed some compassion and sympathy. But now I hide my pain, exhaustion and anguish. I try to act normal. I push myself to the limit of my endurance. And when I reach the limit, I try not to act tired.

And now people do not understand. They say, "Oh, so you finally decided to come to school," or "Boy, I wish I could go to the doctor every Friday and get out of school" and things like that.

If they only knew. I laugh and joke about it when they say these things, but if they only knew the pain in my heart when they say these things. My friends see me in bed reading or listening to a record. They must think that is all. If only they knew how it hurts to breathe or even just move. If only they knew what it really is like going down to Los Angeles every week. They don't know how much I would rather be in school.

Would they be more sympathetic and understanding if I showed how I really felt? It would be pitiful if I did. As I write this my chest feels as if it is pierced with spikes. Every breath is torture. When I cough, I nearly suffocate in the painful spasm. My back aches and I am exhausted. I don't have the strength to express my pain if I wanted to.

Why must they be vindictive and condemning? If they only knew.

I was upset by this and showed it to Dr. Williams without telling Scott. "He never tells us that this is how he feels, Dr. Williams," I said.

"I think Scott is like a volcano," he told me comfortingly. "He erupts through his writings. It relieves a little of the pressure."

It was around this time that Scott told David, one of his friends, "I could die from what I have." He said he had been reading about Hodgkin's a lot and that people usually died when they were as sick as he was.

"I don't think I'm going to make it," Scott said.

"You'll make it," David reassured him.

"I don't know," Scott said doubtfully. "The doctor asked me to write about how I feel. There is a new medi-

cine they might try on me. If it works, I might make
it."

He had to have the biopsy, however, before Dr. Williams could prescribe the new drug. And before the
biopsy, we had planned to go to Lake Arrowhead with a
group of friends. Scott was looking forward to it, although his back was hurting so much that he told me he
might just stay inside when we got there and enjoy the
scenery instead of going hiking. On the morning we left,
he was in agonizing pain, but he did not say a word about
it. I only learned of his pain later when I read his green
notebook.

> February 27, 1976 (2:00 a.m.)—This is it. The last
> straw. I am at the breaking point, one thin line from
> losing my sanity. At any moment I expect to break. I
> just have had it. I don't know what happens next.
> Maybe the torture of more treatment. Maybe worse. I
> might die. Which I would much rather do. I know what
> will happen when I die. I don't know what will happen
> after my operation. I may get complications and have a
> long drawn out torturous stay.
>
> Why can't I just be normal like everyone else? Why
> can't I just run—and not fall down, gasping for breath,
> my sides and head throbbing with pain? I want to hike,
> work, go to school, have fun. Damn, I can't even play
> with my dog without getting tired! I would give any-
> thing just to be well. I just want it to end.

But as we left for Lake Arrowhead that morning, Scott
gave no hint of his feelings—either his pain or his despair.
He protected us from the hurt of knowing how he felt,
what he thought.

The house at Lake Arrowhead was full. Our friends,
the Zells, and their three children got there a couple of
hours after we did. And then the Fauvers arrived—all six

of them. Nine children and six adults. Lots of chatter, laughter, and fun. And Scott did not just sit in the house and admire the scenery. He and Steven and Jeff Fauver went out exploring the mountain trails, which were still covered with snow. And Scott was full of mischief.

At two in the morning, Joanna Zell heard noises. She got up to find Brian, six, and Kenny, three, getting dressed.

"What in the world are you two doing?" she asked sleepily.

"Getting ready to go on our hike with Daddy."

"It's two o'clock in the morning," their mother said. "Get back to bed."

"No, it's not," Brian said. "Scott told us it was six and time to get up." The two boys had woken when Scott got up for water to take a pain pill. When they asked him what he was doing, he said he was getting up and that they had better go wake their daddy or they would be late getting started on their hike.

Brian and Kenny refused to believe their mother when she said it was only two. "It's six, Mommy. Scott said it was six, Mommy," I heard them say.

"I don't care what Scott said," Joanna told them. "Get back in your pajamas and go to bed. Daddy will wake you up when it's time for your hike."

Ronnie was awake now, too, and I told him what had been going on. The two of us smothered our laughter under the covers and hoped that Joanna would speak to us in the morning.

It was a good weekend. Good friends. A happy time. We drove back Sunday, and Monday morning, Scott and I drove down to Los Angeles. And he was admitted to Childrens once again.

Chapter Sixteen

Scott was a veteran of Childrens Hospital by now. He knew how everything worked—and didn't work. He knew about the inefficiencies and blunders of the system. While Dr. Williams was examining him after he had been admitted to Childrens this time, Scott told him that his back hurt and asked for a prescription for pain pills. He knew that the nurses could not give him pain pills without an order from the doctor. And he knew that his back was going to hurt even more later in the day. That was the pattern of his backaches.

"I have some of his pain pills with me," I said.

"Fine. Give Scott one now," said Dr. Williams, "and I'll write an order for more."

> March 2, 1976 (midnight)—So this is how they run this hospital now. Well, whoever introduced this routine can shove it up their descending colon. The medicine nurse distributes medication. If he or she is at the other end of the hall, I must wait until he gets to my room to place my order. Then he gets the medicine and returns in anywhere from fifteen minutes to several hours.

Today I got a backache before dinner. Mom ordered a pain pill at quarter past six. The nurse told us that the medicine nurse was out to dinner. The rules, of course, prohibit any other nurse from giving me medicine. Mom and I went to eat in the cafeteria, but I had too much pain to eat. We saw the medicine nurse in the cafeteria. He was sitting and talking.

I went back to my room where a nurse chewed me out for not eating anything. I told her I was in too much pain, but she didn't listen. Just kept on chewing me out. Mom asked one of the nurses again for my pain pill. The nurse left, returned and said the medicine nurse had already given it to me. The medicine nurse had signed that he had given me the pill. They could not give me one until he returned and confirmed that he had *not* given me a pill. I got my pill at half past seven, by which time I was writhing in pain and very perturbed.

I felt guilty that I was not more aggressive in seeing that Scott was taken care of. It was easy for me to wait patiently. I was not in pain. Every time I asked at the nurses' desk for a pain pill or anything else for Scott, I felt guilty for bothering them. And they usually treated my requests with a certain impatience. So I'd return to Scott and tell him that the doctor or nurse would be in soon. He would get mad at me and keep after me to check again.

I told Mary Anderson, the head of public relations who had become a friend, that I did not like to complain, but that I was often ashamed because I was not more aggressive in Scott's behalf. "It seems to be the pattern that a lot of parents follow," she said. "You find yourself in a frightening situation and think that if you just don't disrupt the system, everything will go all right." And that was exactly how I felt.

Scott often felt he was at the mercy of bunglers or

worse. And I could not blame him. When I arrived the next morning, Scott said, "Guess what happened last night?

"After you left, Dr. Woolley's assistant came in to examine me and he told me my surgery was scheduled for this morning. I told him it wasn't until Thursday, but he said that it was written on his schedule that I was to have a neck biopsy this morning.

"I told him I had to have a transfusion first because I was anemic. And a lymphangiogram so they would know which node they wanted to take out. But he wouldn't believe me."

I was horrified. "What happened?"

"I finally convinced him to call and check. And the records showed that I was due for tests before surgery. But I was scared! I thought I was going to have to have the surgery anyway, just because the doctor had it written down."

The next morning Scott had his lymphangiogram. His first one had been a traumatic experience and he dreaded having another, but the doctor had told him that a new injection now made it possible to do one without having to cut his foot open to insert the dye. All they had to do was give him an injection between the first and second toes of each foot.

As I walked down the corridor toward the Nuclear Medicine unit, I heard a loud, steady moaning. One of Scott's doctors was standing outside the door. He was looking at me strangely. And at that very moment, I understood why. That was Scott moaning!

"Is that Scott?" I asked foolishly.

The doctor nodded and put his arm around me, as we walked into the room where another doctor was giving Scott his second injection. One of the aides was saying, "Scream if you want, but just hold still."

The doctor pulled the needle from between Scott's

toes and said, "It's finished. It's all over. You did a good job of holding still." He patted Scott on the leg and left the room.

When I saw Dr. Williams later that morning, I said, "I found a will on Scott's clipboard this morning. He must have written it last night. It's very detailed. He's left most everything to Steven. I forget what he left to me."

"He's probably going to leave you old Dr. Williams," he laughed. Then he became very serious. "Is Scott worried about his surgery tomorrow?"

"I didn't think so, but now—well, he may be more worried than he lets on."

Dr. Williams nodded with his eyes closed in the understanding way that had become familiar to me by now. "I'll drop by later and talk to him." He started down the corridor, then turned and came back. "Elaine, how about you? Are you worried about his surgery?"

"A little," I said. "I'm always apprehensive. But I'm sure everything will go all right."

"Good," he said and gave me a hug before he left.

I went back to Scott. Tears were streaming down his cheeks. He opened his eyes, but did not move, as he was supposed to remain perfectly still during the lymphangiogram. "My back is hurting, Mom," he said.

A technician volunteered to go get Scott a pain pill. He came back and said the medicine nurse had promised to come right down with the pill. We waited. Scott lay there like a statue. A statue with tears. The technician asked if his back was worse. "Yes," whispered Scott.

I told the technician about what had happened the night before and how it had taken more than an hour before Scott got his pill. "If the nurse had not given Scott the pill when he did," I said, "I had decided I was going to go to the nurses' desk and tell them I was going to give him one myself."

"Do you have a pill with you now?" he asked.

I nodded.

"Well, why don't you give it to him? I see no reason for this crap of letting someone be in pain when you can do something about it." He gave me a glass of water with a bent glass straw so Scott could drink without moving. And I gave Scott his pill.

Five minutes later, the medicine nurse walked in. The same man who had been on duty the night before. "Here's Scott's medicine," he said.

"I just gave him a pill."

"You what!" he said angrily.

"I just gave Scott his pill. He was crying, the pain was so bad."

"You can't do that," the nurse said. "Where did you get the pill?" he demanded.

"I have the prescription," I told him, "and I was going to tell you about it so you could put the pill on the medicine chart."

"You'd better turn those pain pills in." He was getting increasingly angry with me. Almost threatening. Then the technician, who had busied himself recording Scott's tests, got up and walked over to the nurse. "Buddy, we can solve this problem right now. You know what you can do?"

I held my breath. The nurse was silent.

"Scott's tests are finished," the technician continued. "He's had his pain pill, so you can just put him back in his wheelchair and take him back to his room." I could have hugged him. And even the disgruntled nurse looked relieved.

The surgery went well. They removed Scott's node easily and he was back in his room very shortly afterward. Two days later, he was ready to go home. But before he was released, Dr. Williams took us to one of the little conference rooms for a talk.

"Scott," he said, "the lymph node biopsy was positive.

And the lymphangiogram was abnormal. Especially on your right side."

"Oh," said Scott.

"So when you've recovered from the surgery, we're going to start you on Velban and a new drug to be taken orally along with the prednisone and procarbazine that you've had before."

"You said I'd gain weight on Velban, didn't you?" Scott asked.

"Other patients have. I think you will. So, Scott, you have your mom bring you down in a week and we'll see how you're feeling."

As we got up to leave, Dr. Williams put his arm around Scott's shoulders and drew him aside. "I want to ask you something, Scott," he said. "You've been on so much treatment now. And you know about your tests and the effects of your treatment. What would you think about coming down here this summer and helping us out? You could answer some of the other kids' questions. How's that sound to you?"

Scott gave that big grin of his. "I think I'd kinda like that."

"All right then. That's settled. We'll have you working for us this summer," he said, and gave Scott a pat on the back before he left to write the order for Scott's release papers.

We sat in Scott's room waiting for the papers so we could go home. After fifteen minutes, Scott began nagging Ronnie and me to find out what was taking so long. "They'll call us when the papers are ready," I said. "Just be patient." After an hour had passed, Ronnie went to the desk to see what was holding them up.

"Oh, they've been ready for an hour," the clerk said. "I was waiting for you to come pick them up."

Scott was furious. So was Ronnie. And so was I. We had

been sitting in full sight of the clerk all that time. She could see that Scott was dressed and ready to leave. She could have called us without even having to raise her voice if she did not feel like walking the ten or fifteen feet to the room.

It was just another part of all the annoyances that seemed to be more aggravating every time we went to the hospital. It may have been that, after all these years, Scott was weaker and more impatient and we were more frightened and more fatigued. But it seemed at times as if no one cared that there was a very ill boy who was in pain most of the time and who was anxious and worried.

Chapter Seventeen

EVERY time Scott came home from the hospital, it was cause for rejoicing. But this time was different.

Just one day after he got home, I had to take him to see Dr. Martin in Ventura, because his lungs were congested. But the lung congestion was nothing compared to his back, which hurt all the time now. The pain no longer came and went. It stayed. Scott took pain pills throughout the day and night. He would wake me eight or nine times a night to refill his hot water bottle or rub his back. I felt myself turning grouchy because of lack of sleep, so one night I changed sides of the bed with Ronnie, so that Ronnie would be the one Scott would wake when he came in.

I felt much better after a full night's sleep, but that morning Scott was rude and unpleasant. "Stop talking that way to me," I told him. "I know you don't feel good, but it won't hurt you to be polite."

"Well, you and Dad are grouchy and mean to me."

"When?" I demanded. "Just tell me one time."

"Last night. When I asked Dad for the hot water bottle. He just shoved it at me and called me a pest.

"I can't help it if I'm sick!" he yelled. He got up from the sofa where he had been lying and shouted again, "I can't help it!" and went into his room, slamming the door.

I felt terrible. Feeling sorry for myself because my sleep was interrupted. What was the matter with me? Granted, Ronnie and I had not slept a full night for almost a week, but neither had Scott. And he was ill. And in pain. I went into Scott's room to apologize.

"Get out of here!" he yelled.

I left and went to my own room, threw myself across the bed, and cried. I hated Ronnie for having been so impatient with Scott. And I hated myself for the same reason and for not being more understanding of Scott's feelings. When Ronnie came home that night, I told him what had happened and he went to talk to Scott.

"I'm sorry I hurt your feelings last night," he said.

"Well, I'm sorry if I'm sick. I don't mean to be a pest," Scott answered stiffly, still angry.

"I guess I must have sounded mad, but I wasn't," Ronnie told him. "I was just sleepy. You know, sometimes this is hard on all of us and I want you to know I'm really sorry, Scott."

A few minutes later Scott came out of his room and joined us while we watched television. It was like any other evening. Scott was lying on the floor watching television with Ronnie and Ronnie was massaging his back. The storm was over.

Although I had resolved to be more understanding, I was concerned that he was getting behind in his schoolwork. Scott enjoyed reading about his hobbies and drawing detailed pictures of medals and his latest interest, guns.

"If you're well enough to read and draw guns, you're well enough to do your schoolwork," I would scold. When my mother heard me one day, she said, "Why don't you let Scott do what he wants for a while? He looks like he feels so bad. Let him do the things he enjoys. He can catch up with school later."

I asked Dr. Williams if I should tell Scott it was all right to forget about his schoolwork and concentrate on getting well. "I wouldn't have him quit going to school," he told me. I had not made it clear that Scott had only gone to school two or three days since Christmas. I finally decided I would stop pressuring and let Scott make the decision about how much studying to do. If the new drug worked, we could think about school again.

So I am back on treatment. Now what? What happens next? The first time was inevitable. The second was a shock. But then I did so well. I was almost normal. I was finally confident. This new treatment was the last I would ever need. I *would* make it!

I had hiked the roughest trails in the Sespe, made the Honor Roll at school, created just as much mischief as Steven. I was psychologically jubilant, physically on the road to normality.

Then I got anemic. But I'd get better. Then I caught pneumonia. I was starting to have backaches. But they would go away and I'd be fine. There were no symptoms of disease in me and all the x-rays and bone scans were negative. It was just a bad case of pneumonia or something.

But all I did was get worse. Both physically and mentally. It just couldn't be the disease again. This treatment was doing so well. There just couldn't be another operation. It just couldn't happen or—or—could it?

It just could not be. Anyway, if it was, if this new treatment wasn't working, then what would they put me on? Did they have any other forms? No!

Maybe, maybe this is just—it. Maybe—my time—is up.

But why?

The new treatment was effective. Just a few days after the first one, Scott's backaches started to become less agonizing. And then less frequent. But the next scheduled treatment had to be postponed, because the drugs had lowered his blood count. Scott spent more and more time in his room listening to his records and writing in the green notebook.

March 23, 1976 (at home)—I lie back and my mind becomes part of the music and my emotions dance. My mind howls in agony and wails in the hellish screams and moans of Tchaikovsky's Sixth to come to a quiet depressing end, leaving me to lament. My mind swirling in a dark chaotic whirlpool of depression.

My mind floats happily and carefree on a sea of flowers in a cool green meadow somewhere between the Sierra and insanity while I listen to his Waltz of the Flowers. I am a butterfly, dancing. No, the flowers. The warmth. I am.

Sometimes my interpretations vary with my frame of mind. Almost anything sounds bleak and woeful when I am bleak and woeful. Yet sometimes a piece can lift me out of a mild depression—or throw me with force into the jaws of terror.

You may think why do I let myself become depressed and agonized? Why not just open my eyes? Face reality? Well, I do. But what is reality for me?

Will this new treatment work? It might fail just like last time. Then what? Is it worth it? What is reality? To sit and listen, my mind becoming part of the music itself? I sit barely able to distinguish reality from the unreal.

But—I must accomplish something. So I write my feelings. And all I spew forth are insane, disorganized, mixed-up ravings. I must live a little longer, experience a little more. I must think. Organize my thoughts. Then maybe I can write something creative. Accomplish something.

I *must* live. I want to. Oh, how I want to! But what if I don't? This is the third try. What if I strike out? Again? There are only so many kinds of treatment. I can only take so much.

Death is lurking in the shadows. Behind me always, snatching and grabbing at me.

Some day I fear
My body, tired, aching, sore to the bone . . .
Death will snatch.

I will not pull away.
                    I will lie back.
     I will claim my rest, for I have fought a hard battle
                    and the end has finally come.

March 24, 1976—Oh, the despair! My mind is in a vise of anxiety, despair, anger. Twisted between thoughts of imminent death and the want to live. I am elated one moment, finally convinced I will live, get better. I'll swim, hike, see the country day in and day out. Free of pain!

And then I realize it was for but a brief period.

I seem to be filled to the bursting point with pent-up anguish, pain, *fear!*

If I would scream, venting my frustration through my scarred, pneumonia-filled, dilapidated lungs, the mountains would tremble, the creeks stop flowing. The summer air would frost. The trees would shed their leaves. And the land would weep.

I sometimes want to crawl away and die amidst the country I love. There is barely any strength left in my body or soul to fight the battle I must fight. Never pausing, not able to stop and rest. It is such a tiring, painful battle for me to simply survive.

I am so tired. My body aches so. I want just a little rest, but no. I must hurry. The struggle never ends, the fight continues without pause.

Some day the battle will end. I will conquer or die. Either way is fine with me. I am tired. I want to rest.

On April 3, Scott called me at the store late in the afternoon. "Mom, can you buy a new thermometer. I just broke ours trying to take my temperature. I feel really hot."

I rushed home with a new thermometer. His temperature was 103 and he ached all over. I gave him two Tylenol and put him in a lukewarm tub. And for the next twenty-four hours, we controlled his fever with Tylenol and lukewarm baths, sponge baths when he was too weak to step into the tub.

A couple of days later, I took him to Ventura for his blood test. Dr. Martin reported that Scott's hemoglobin was down. It was 6.7. His platelets were down, too. "I think you should call Dr. Williams," he said, "and see if he wants Scott to have a transfusion before his Friday appointment in Los Angeles. Tell him I don't see any immediate danger. I just think he should be informed." Dr. Williams said he thought we might just as well wait until Scott came down to Childrens in three days. That afternoon, Scott said, "My throat hurts. I feel like there is something in it." And he began to cry. I was frightened. Scott rarely cried.

On Friday he was feeling miserable. He lay down in the back seat during our drive to Childrens, and when we got there, he said, "Mom, can you get me a wheelchair? I'm too tired to walk."

Steven was with us this day and took over as "driver" for Scott in the wheelchair. One of Scott's doctors, Dr. Hoffman, stopped us in the hall and asked, "How are you feeling today, Scott?"

Scott looked up and with a small smile replied, "Guess."

Dr. Hoffman nodded and said, "Feel pretty lousy, eh?"

The doctor guessed correctly, but as lousy as Scott felt he still found strength to smile and tease with Steven who was doing his best to cheer Scott up.

As we neared the elevators and escalators, Steven asked Scott, "Which do you want to take—the elevator or escalators?"

"The escalators are faster, you don't have to wait for them," Scott answered mischievously.

"Okay," said Steven as he wheeled Scott toward the escalators.

"Oh no you don't. Steven, bring him back here!" I yelled.

They returned, both displaying big grins, discussing how much more fun a ride on the escalator would have been with a wheelchair.

Later, when Dr. Williams examined him, he did not mention the wheelchair although it seemed to take up most of the examining room. He left for a moment and came back with Dr. Hoffman who began examining Scott. As he was feeling Scott's abdomen, Dr. Williams said, "Do you feel that?" Dr. Hoffman nodded.

"Have you been bruising much?" he asked Scott.

"Not much. A few small bruises on my legs. And I had a nosebleed a week or so ago."

"Bad?"

"No, a light one."

"How about your gums. Do they bleed when you brush your teeth?"

"Only when I use a wire toothbrush," Scott said, smiling.

There were more questions. Finally Dr. Williams said, "Scott's X rays show changes in his lungs. And his liver is enlarged. His blood cells are showing changes, too."

"What kind of changes?" I asked.

"We're seeing leukemic properties."

Leukemia! It was too much for Scott. He began to cry. Very softly. No one said anything.

Dr. Williams broke the silence. "I think what we'll have to do is admit Scott and start a transfusion. I'd like to run more blood tests and X rays. And do a bone marrow. If you can stay here, we can start the transfusion tonight."

"We can stay," I said.

But Scott had gotten himself under control and he pleaded, "Can't we wait a few days? Can't I go home for the weekend?"

"Well, let me go call Dr. Martin and see what he says," Dr. Williams answered and left the room. I wondered why he would have to ask Dr. Martin. Later I learned he was simply calling him to tell him what was happening.

He came back soon. "I've talked to Dr. Martin and he told me not to let you talk me out of it, Scott. But I tell you what. I think we can let you go home tonight if you promise to come back Sunday afternoon."

"I promise," Scott said eagerly.

We helped Scott back into the wheelchair and I helped him stretch out in the back seat of the car. As I drove off, I caught a glimpse of the wheelchair in my rearview mirror. Standing there empty. And I shivered.

Chapter Eighteen

WHEN we got back from Los Angeles that Friday, Scott was terribly depressed. He was in such pain that he hardly slept that night. The next day, he made it to the living room sofa in his pajamas, where he watched television and dozed now and then when the pain pills gave him a few moments surcease.

All I could think of were those two words—leukemic properties. I was distressed that Dr. Williams had said them in front of Scott. Most of the doctors at Childrens believed it was important to be honest with their young patients. And I know I would want to know what I had. But still—I wished Scott had not had to hear this.

That night Scott slept with Ronnie and me in our bed. We took turns rubbing his aching joints and sponging him with a wet washcloth. Twice, when his fever went over 103 degrees, we put him in the tub. "You just have the flu," I remember telling him. "It's harder on you because your blood count is so low." I told him this so many times that I ended up believing it.

It was a relief when Sunday morning came and I could think about preparing to go back to Childrens. A relief for Ronnie and me, that is. Scott was full of dread.

"Will they do the bone marrow today?" I reminded him that Dr. Williams had said it would probably be Monday or Tuesday.

"Mom, I just don't want to have a bone marrow."

"I know, Scott. I really know. But they have to find out why your hemoglobin is so low."

"Promise me, Mom, that you won't let them do it unless they put me out. Don't sign for it unless they promise."

I promised.

It was a beautiful spring day, warm and sunny. We were driving along Scott's favorite stretch of road beside the Santa Clara River when he said, "I'm going to be sick," and grabbed the pan that we always kept in the car. When he was through, I took the pan to empty it, but first I showed the contents to Ronnie.

"Look, doesn't that look like coffee grounds?"

He nodded.

"That means he's vomiting blood."

As we started up again, Scott said, "You know, Mom, your stomach is lined with blood. And since I'm low on platelets, that's why blood came up when I threw up." That made me feel better. I told myself that all he needed was a transfusion.

We arrived at one, but we had to wait almost an hour before our name was called by the admitting clerk. Scott was sitting in a wheelchair, full of pain and so weak that he could barely hold his head up, but when the clerk finally called us and I started to sign the papers, he warned, "Watch what you sign, Mom."

They were the standard admitting forms. I did not read them. I knew what they said.

"Mom," Scott cried in distress as I signed, "you didn't read what you signed. Are you sure you didn't sign for a bone marrow?"

I reassured him that I had not signed for any surgical procedure.

An hour or so after Scott was finally in his room being examined by a young intern, Dr. Johnson, Dr. Hoffman came in. "Scott is very sick," he said to Ronnie and me. "He's very ill. I'm quite concerned. His heart is working very hard. I'm worried about that."

What was he saying? And why was he saying it in front of Scott? What possessed the man? Did he think that Scott could not hear him? And what effect would these remarks have on Scott? The doctor's words, swift and deadly, threw terror into Ronnie and me.

He led us to a conference room where he began again: "I'm quite worried about Scott. He's in critical condition. His hemoglobin is low. His heart is having to work very hard. He may go into heart failure."

And then he added, "He may not make it through the night."

Yes, he will! Yes, he will! I shouted silently.

Dr. Hoffman got up and walked to the blackboard on the wall. "We have been trying to figure out what has been causing Scott's low hemoglobin for months. Now we think we know. We think it's a rare type of leukemia that starts from a blood cell." He drew a picture of the cell structure on the blackboard as Ronnie and I sat there stunned.

"This type of leukemia is always fatal. Sometimes the only treatment required is transfusions. Many patients have been kept under control with transfusions for as long as five years. We'll be doing the bone marrow tomorrow and some other tests. Tonight, we hope that some oxygen and red blood cells will help him feel better. My main concern is that he could go into heart failure any minute."

It is true what they say about hating people who bring

bad news. I hated Dr. Hoffman at that moment, as he calmly, almost casually, told us all this. And then I prayed. I prayed that Scott would live through the night. Please, God. Through this night. And suddenly I became calm. The hate disappeared. I knew Scott would be all right that night. And he was.

In the morning, he began worrying about the bone marrow again. "Did you ask them to put me out?"

"Yes," I told him. "Dr. Hoffman said they could tranquilize you very heavily."

"Please make sure they do, Mom," he said weakly. "I hurt so bad all over as it is." Dr. McCallister, whom Scott knew from his clinic visits, had told me, "What we'll do is put a tranquilizer in his IV and give him a pain pill along with an anesthetic patch over the bone-marrow area. That's all we can do. It's impossible to anesthetize the bone. But this should make it as easy as possible."

An hour went by. Crept by. Scott's worries were mounting. And so were mine. I kept praying. Praying that it was not really leukemia. Please, God. Not leukemia. Finally a nurse came to put the tranquilizer in the IV and gave Scott a pain pill. She applied the anesthetic patch. And a few minutes later, Dr. Johnson and Dr. McCallister arrived to do the bone marrow.

"Scott, do you want me to wait outside or stay with you?" I asked.

"You can stay if you want."

All I wanted to do, seeing the fear in Scott's eyes, was pick him up in my arms and run away with him. There had been pain in Scott's eyes for years now. But never fear. And the fear was dreadful.

They started the bone marrow. Swabbed on antiseptic.

"Are you sure the needle is sharp?" Scott asked.

"Yes," said Dr. Johnson. He began to thrust the big hollow needle into Scott's hipbone. Then inserted the syringe needle inside the hollow needle. He pulled on the syringe. No marrow.

"You'll have to try deeper," Dr. McCallister said. Dr. Johnson pulled out the small needle and worked the hollow needle deeper into Scott's bone and tried again. He pulled and pulled on the syringe trying to get enough marrow for the test. It was half an hour before he was through. As Dr. McCallister left, he told me he was taking the marrow to the lab and would let me know the results as soon as possible.

When he came back that afternoon, he told me they had not been able to get any results. They would have to do another the next day. "It often happens that we have to do several before we can read results," he said.

Scott only smiled once that day. Tom Collins, the young man in charge of the recreation room, brought the pet guinea pig in to Scott who cuddled and stroked him for a few minutes. He had a tender smile on his lips as he held the soft, furry animal.

The next morning, Scott said, "Mom, you know the red-haired nurse? She came in last night and gave me a back rub. She asked if I said prayers at night and I said yes. So she asked if she could pray with me. We said a prayer together. It made me feel better."

I was grateful for this kindness. I could not pray with Scott. I was afraid he would get the idea that prayer was all that was left and refuse to have any more tests or treatments. So I prayed silently day and night for God to guide the doctors or perform a miracle. I was grateful that the red-haired nurse had done what I could not do.

The second bone marrow was even more grueling than the first. It took forty-five minutes and five attempts before they got enough for the test. A little later, Dr. Johnson came in to get blood.

"I need two samples, Scott," he said.

"Can't you get it all in one stick?"

"No. We need one from your vein and another from an artery so we can measure the oxygen in your blood."

No sooner had he taken his two samples when Dr. McCallister came rushing in. "Have you drawn his blood yet? We need some more."

Later, Dr. McCallister reported that they had not been able to get results from the second bone-marrow test. "This often happens when cells are multiplying fast and are packed," he told me.

"Does this mean he has leukemia?" I was afraid to ask, but I had to.

"We're sure he does," the doctor said. "We're just trying to pin down exactly what kind."

Late that afternoon, Dr. Williams came by and asked Ronnie and me to come talk with him in the conference room. The blackboard still held the sketches Dr. Hoffman had made.

"Scott's chest X rays are showing changes," Dr. Williams said. "We are not sure what they mean. They may be from his disease or pneumonia or some other cause."

"Does Scott have leukemia?" I asked the question again. I still could not accept what the other doctor had told me earlier.

Dr. Williams nodded.

"When did it start?"

"We don't know. We've been trying to pin down the cause of his low hemoglobin for months now. We found two antibodies, but we were not sure that was the cause. His bone marrow in the fall was negative. We just can't say exactly when it started."

I had something more on my mind. "Dr. Williams, it just made me sick when you told me in front of Scott that his blood tests were showing leukemic properties. Do we have to tell Scott that he has leukemia?"

"Yes," he said bluntly.

"Why?"

"We can't keep this from him. He will know without our telling him."

I thought about how careful I had been not to tell Scott that Hodgkin's disease was cancer—and how he had known it all the time. I did not want to agree with Dr. Williams, but I knew he was right.

"Dr. Hoffman told us that some patients with leukemia can live for five years with transfusions. I guess we'll have to learn to live with this and hope for a new drug—or a miracle."

Dr. Williams spoke gently and slowly, looking into my eyes. "Elaine, if Scott does not respond to treatment or you do not get your miracle, he could have as little as three months."

Don't listen, heart! Those are just words, I told myself. "You mean you would accept a miracle?" I asked.

Dr. Williams gave a little smile. "Yes, I would accept a miracle." Months later I thought how hard this must be on doctors. Not only do they suffer defeat against disease, but they have to tell the parents and face their disbelief, their grief, their shock.

Each day Scott had become increasingly drowsy. This bothered him. "You said when my fever went down, I wouldn't feel so sleepy," he said, "but I still do."

"They've been giving you stronger medication for your aches. That probably is doing it," I told him. Just then a nurse came in the room with more medicine. "Is this what's making me so sleepy?" Scott asked. "Oh, no," she said, "there's nothing in this that would make you sleepy."

"Mom, what is it? What's making me so sleepy?" he asked in distress.

I had no answer now.

And so Scott took it upon himself to apologize to his visitors for his drowsiness.

To his beloved Grandpa Harry and Grandma Christine who came in the afternoons and relieved me by taking turns rubbing Scott's legs and back.

To his Aunt Phyllis as he asked her to apply pressure to his arms after his blood tests, "because that will save my veins." Phyllis brought cards from Mark and Kym, and once Scott awoke suddenly and asked her to get a pencil and said, "Write—to Kym, Hello—Love, Scott."

When Scott apologized to Carolyn LaPorte who made a surprise visit Wednesday evening, Carolyn said, "That's all right, Scott," as she rose to leave, "I just want you to know that I'm praying for you and that I love you."

"I love you too," Scott answered, then he turned toward me and said, "I love both of you."

Scott had been admitted to the hospital on Sunday. On Thursday morning, he woke up and said he would like some cereal. This was the most encouraging development so far. I flew to get the nurse. He hadn't been eating at all. Soon a tray came with cereal and milk. The nurse and I propped Scott up in bed and he tried to eat.

But he kept missing his mouth. The cereal and milk would slide off his spoon and dribble down the front of his pajamas. He refused to let me help him and went on weakly stabbing his spoon into the cereal and then not being able to get it into his mouth. My heart was breaking.

Ronnie and Steven drove down from Fillmore that evening with cards and presents from Scott's friends. Scott just looked blankly as we showed him each present and read the cards to him. Finally he said, "Tell everyone thanks," and fell asleep.

Ronnie and I went to talk with Dr. McCallister. Why

were so many things going wrong? Had they learned any-thing more? "I've just finished talking to Dr. Williams," he said. "He's ordered more blood tests. And we're going to run a forty-eight-hour urine culture. But right now, we don't have any answers." He turned toward Scott's room and shook his clenched fist in the air. He was as frustrated as we were.

Dr. Johnson came in to draw more blood. He had to go deep to reach an artery. When they pulled the needle from Scott's arm, Scott looked at me and pleaded, "Oh, Mom. Please. Don't let them stick me anymore."

I leaned over and kissed him and told him I loved him. I could not make a promise that I could not keep. I told him that I was going home with Steven that night, but that his dad was going to stay with him. He nodded. Ronnie sat beside Scott all night, swabbing his blistered lips with glycerine and rubbing his aching body.

Twice Scott asked him, "Dad, am I going to die?" Both times Ronnie said, "No, Scott, you're going to be all right."

Chapter Nineteen

THE NEXT morning I was getting ready to drive back to the hospital when the telephone rang. It was Ronnie. Scott had been moved to Intensive Care. I should get there as soon as possible. Scott was having trouble with his breathing.

I forgot about speed limits as I drove to Los Angeles, and when I arrived at the hospital, I ran from the parking lot and along the corridors to Intensive Care. I knocked on the door. A nurse let me in. There was Ronnie standing beside Scott's bed. Scott had a heart monitor taped to him, an oxygen mask on his face, platelets were running through his IV, and Dr. Johnson was preparing to insert another tube.

My first thought was how beautiful he looked. His face was no longer swollen and distorted, but his struggles for breath proved to me that he was in trouble.

Dr. Williams was there looking at X rays with two hematologists. He led me to a little room where he told me that Scott was "critical." I wanted to deny it. But it was true. I knew it.

We went back. Dr. Johnson was preparing to insert a catheter, telling Scott what he was doing. "No, no!" Scott cried and tried to push the doctor away. I held his arms while the doctor went ahead. Dr. McCallister came and took blood from an artery deep in Scott's arm. I could hear Scott pleading with me the night before, not to let them stick him anymore. But I had to let them. I had to let them do everything they could to save him so I watched as they stuck him once more. A cardiologist came in and started listening to his heart.

The inhalation therapist bent over Scott and told him that he was going to give him extra oxygen to help him breathe. Scott did not answer. After the doctor had drawn blood from his artery, a wide, unseeing stare had come on his face.

An aide called my parents and asked them to come and to bring Steven. Dr. Williams asked Ronnie and me to come with him. We went to the little room again. Dr. Johnson and Dr. McCallister joined us there.

"Scott is in very critical condition. His liver and kidneys are not functioning. His white count has gone off the scale. His hemoglobin is very, very low. He is bleeding internally. He's not getting enough oxygen, and his heart is working harder and harder trying to keep up."

Dr. Williams paused.

Ronnie and I knew what was coming. Other mothers had told me of similar conversations with Dr. Williams. "I think what we're going to have to decide now is whether or not to put Scott on a heart machine. His heart is not going to keep up much longer. We have to ask you now—do you want us to put him on the heart machine if his heart stops?"

"No. No machines," Ronnie said decisively.

"Wait a minute, Ronnie," I said in panic, "we've got to make sure we make the right decision." I still did not believe that Scott was dying. Everyone's face and actions seemed to show this as an accepted fact and I acted as if I were accepting it too, but I think I was more stunned than accepting. Scott was alive. There was still time for a miracle. Please, God, make it soon, I pleaded silently with all my heart.

I turned to Dr. Williams. I was going to ask him what he would do if Scott were his child. But I couldn't. We had to make this decision ourselves. I turned to Dr. McCallister. "You've heard what Dr. Williams told us. What do you think?"

"Scott's disease has spread," he said quietly. "He has leukemia with apparent involvement of his major organs. I think the heart machine would prolong his present condition without improving it."

I hated this answer. But he was honest. I recognized this.

I turned to Dr. Johnson. "What do you think?"

"If this were an accident case where we had to keep Scott's heart going while we did some repair work, I'd recommend it. But Scott has many problems that can't be repaired," he answered gently.

The decision had to be made. I had not imagined it would come like this. I had thought there would be time for prayer and meditation. But this was nothing imagined. This was real life. Real death.

We'd had all the facts explained quickly and kindly. I knew Ronnie's feelings, but I also knew that he would let me make the final decision. I took one last slow look at the doctors' faces, then stared at my clenched hands and said, "Well, if God does not want to perform a miracle and completely heal him now," I sighed, nodded my head, and said it, "we'll let him go."

We were all silent for a few seconds—a chapel could not have been as reverent. Dr. Williams put his arm around me as I started to cry. After a few seconds, I turned and reached for Ronnie. He was holding his head in his hands and fighting his tears.

"We've had four and a half good years," he said, his voice cracking.

"We've had fifteen and a half wonderful years," I said, with a new determination that stopped my tears. "Now, please, let's get back to Scott.

"Steven is coming down," I told Dr. Williams. "Can he see Scott?"

He held both my hands. "As soon as Steven gets here, have me paged and I'll talk to him first."

Ronnie was at Scott's side, holding his hand. I stood beside him and kissed his forehead. "Dad and Mom are here, Scott. We love you. It's going to be all right. Just rest."

"Water," he rasped. The nurse heard him, but made no move toward giving him water since they were trying to limit his intake. So I just kissed him again. He asked for water several times in that rasping voice. I felt so helpless. Then Scott turned toward me and opened his eyes wide as if he were trying to focus on my face. I bent over and said, "You're doing fine, baby. Everything's okay."

Steven and Dr. Williams came in to see Scott. Dr. Williams had his arm around Steven as he said, "Steven offered to give blood for Scott if that would help him." He looked at Steven, then at me and continued, "I told Steve that would not be necessary right now, but if we need blood from him, we'll let him know." Dr. Williams left for a moment after Steven was seated in a chair near Scott's side.

Later my parents came in. Ronnie and I sat by Scott. There was a change of nurses. We stayed, never taking our eyes from our son.

"Is this my world?" Scott said unexpectedly. The words came slowly, painfully in that rasping voice.

"What did you say, honey?" I asked, startled.

"Is this my world?" he asked again, struggling back from unconsciousness. He was on the threshold. Wavering between life and death. Almost into the next world. Bewildered.

"Yes, Scott, this is your world. You're here in the hospital with Mom and Dad. Steven's here, too." Steven grasped Scott's shoulder, his eyes filling with tears. I stood next to Scott, embracing him as best I could, and whispered what I hoped was a comforting prayer in his ear.

The doctors and nurses moved in as if on one breath, one impulse. They touched. Checked. Explored my son's body. The nurse removed Scott's oxygen mask. And then they fell back.

Scott took two more breaths.

The computer lights above his bed danced—and fell still.

And that was all.

Death had entered the room as Scott spoke. Entered Scott's body. Released him. His suffering was over. This was his world no longer, and as I kissed his eyes, his mouth, his needle-scarred arms and hands, I knew that he was in another world now. A world without suffering. A world of joy. A world without end.

It was five minutes of three on April 16, 1976. It was Good Friday.

Chapter Twenty

SCOTT was gone. And we were left with our grief. In the days, weeks, and months after Scott's death, Steven and Ronnie and I suffered in our own ways. I was beset not only by sorrow, but by guilt. I kept wondering— had we done everything we could for Scott? Did we say and do the right things? Could we have made life easier for him? And, most tormenting of all, did I possibly make it harder for him? These questions chased through my mind night after sleepless night, day after grieving day.

And then Scott gave me an answer.

Going through his papers—and there were many I had not read, papers that he had tucked away in his desk and bureau drawers—I found one headed "How I Would Show Love."

How I would show love is by being thoughtful and caring, helping in any way I could. I think the best way to show it is to say "I love you." Hugging and kissing would be a nice way too. Laughing and smiling when someone you love is happy and being reassuring and extra, extra kind when the one you love is sad are two very good ways of showing someone you love them.

> Holding hands is a good way to show love. When you
> are very sick, it helps to have someone hold your hand,
> letting the glowing warmth of their love for you trickle
> into you.

I read this over and over. It was as if Scott was showing
his love for us by letting us know that he had felt our love
for him.

I will never stop missing Scott, never stop wanting him
back. There had been times during his illness when I was
tired and despairing and found the strain on the family
almost more than I could handle, but I learned that the
problems of coping with long-term catastrophic illness
were nothing compared to those of facing life without
Scott. I wanted Scott back, even if it meant Scott still
going to the clinic for his checkups and his hated treatments. I told Dr. Williams that I wished Scott could have
lived longer, because I was sure there would be a medical
breakthrough that would cure him. I only dared wish
this, I said, because I thought that although Scott had
suffered, he had not suffered as much as some others.

Dr. Williams shook his head. "Elaine," he said softly,
"I think his writings show us that he suffered a great deal
more than we knew." A few days after this, I found a
poem among Scott's papers that underlined the truth of
Dr. Williams's words.

> I fight courageously, never giving up,
> Never ending fighting.
> Fighting. Losing.
> Going down in battle. Losing.
> Dying
> Courageously.
>
> Dying. Why?
> My struggle so valiant, brave.

Why?
Dying, but still fighting.
Dying, but never giving up.
Why?
So brave was the battle.
Why?

Proudly, majestically, I leave.
Happy, content, I leave.
I have done what I could to the end
Never surrendering.
I leave.
I leave forever.

This was written a year and a half before Scott died. I realized as I read it how much of his pain Scott had kept to himself to protect us. How much the thought of death must have been with him for long months when we never suspected it was his heart's companion.

Webb had told Scott once, "I can stand anything for three days." When I asked Scott what happened after the three days and the pain was still there, he smiled. "I guess you start the three days over again," he said. I have no idea how many times Scott had to start those three days over again. I only know that it was more often than I had ever dreamed.

After Scott's death, my faith in God was even more severely shaken than it had been during his illness. I still prayed. I asked God to cherish my son in heaven. But there were days and nights when I was swept by storms of tears, by doubts, by anger. When I felt that God was cruel. When I even doubted His existence. One day sitting in Scott's room where I spent many hours mourning him, I picked up the green notebook in which he had written for Dr. Williams. A few days before Scott died, he had asked Ronnie to tear the pages out of the notebook and bring them to Los Angeles. Ronnie had done this, and Scott had given the pages to Dr. Williams who later gave them to us. I flipped through the remaining blank pages in the notebook and came upon one with writing.

> God has chosen me, for what I know not.
> Through pain, privation and agony I have suffr'd.
> The reason I know not why.
> Through doubts and temptations I have been
> Unwavering in my faith, clinging to it, my only hope.
>
> Tired now of pain, strife and sorrow,
> I seek rest, the prize that is mine.
> I fear not death, for death is peace and rest.
> Death ushers in a new life for all who believe,
> A life free of pain, sorrow and strife,
> A wonderful gift from our merciful God.
>
> Be not sorrowful when I die.
> I have fought a hard, bitter battle.
> The prize of rest is mine,
> Earned through pain and strife.
> Be not sad, for the prize of peace is finally mine.

This last message from Scott restored my faith. I prayed to be forgiven for my doubts. God had allowed Scott to answer my questions through his poem. God had allowed Scott to ease my torments of guilt. God exists and Scott is with Him.

Many months after Scott died, I stumbled going up the steps of our front porch. I reached out to steady myself. At the very spot where I placed my hand, I saw for the first time a tiny penciled scrawl on the white-painted column. Three little words: "Scott was here."

And that is what is important. Scott *was* here and he left us a legacy of love and courage. I have written this book in an attempt to share that legacy with others. This is what Scott would have wanted.

Appendix

SCOTT made many friends in the hospital, among them a charming and intelligent young woman, Connie Mayer, who is now Connie Mayer Kalter. She was working toward a doctorate in educational psychology and spent one day a week with young patients in the Hematology-Oncology Clinic or on Four West with children suffering from catastrophic diseases—usually cancer. Connie had been impressed with Scott and spent many hours talking with him. And Scott liked Connie very much. During those last days at Childrens, she sat with Scott one night massaging his aching joints and keeping him company.

After Scott died, Connie wrote us a letter telling us what he had meant to her.

> In the 26 years of my life, there have been so few people, public figures or people I've known personally, whom I could truly call heroic. Your son, Scott, was and always will be, heroic to me. In a world where there is so much selfishness and greed, Scott was a shining ray of sunlight in a cloudy sky. It was one of the greatest privileges of my life to have known Scott.

I remember so clearly my first day at Childrens Hospital when I met Scott. I was amazed at his intellectual brilliance, but even more striking was what an exceptional human being he was. To see that kind of goodness and kindness in a person of any age is truly rare. I learned so much from Scott on those Fridays when he would bring his books and fossils and explain things to me. But the greatest lesson I learned from Scott was the way he chose to respond to life. In the midst of sickness, he had such great courage, he was always concerned with the feelings of others, always kind, always courteous, never complained and never lost his sense of humor.

I am so grateful to you for allowing me to see him last Tuesday. I will never forget those hours I spent with him and the things he said to me while he was awake. In the midst of the excruciating pain, he was so selfless. His words were words of concern for the feelings of those around him. To witness that kind of heroism is truly rare in one's lifetime.

He lived his life and approached his death with a courage, bravery and unselfishness that has taught me and all of those who were blessed to know him very much about the meaning of life. He is an example for us all of the highest and most noble that a human being can become.

Thank you for bringing into this world a child who touched my life in a way that will be with me always.

Connie wrote something else that would have pleased Scott even more. Several months after his death, she wrote a paper for her class in Adolescent Development. Its title: "Terminal Illness and the Adolescent." Her professor gave her an A and commented, "Excellent paper. I believe you could develop this for publication." With Connie's permission, I have included her paper in Scott's book. Scott wanted so much to accomplish something in his life. I think he would have been very pleased with this accomplishment, to know that his friend Connie found a meaning in his life and death that could help doctors and nurses and parents help other young people who are suffering from one of the killer diseases. In the last few paragraphs of her paper, she wrote of her experience with Scott and of the night she spent with him before his death. "There was a sense of peace emanating from Scott," she wrote, "which filled me with a mixture of serenity and sadness . . . His family helped him in the difficult task of finding meaning in his suffering."

Perhaps Connie's paper will help other mothers and fathers of dying children to face their death just a little more easily by finding meaning in both life and death. Here is Connie's paper:

Adolescence, even under optimal circumstances, presents some of the most difficult tasks that an individual must face in his lifetime. The early adolescent has recently emerged from the latency period of childhood which is usually characterized by gradual changes and a certain degree of regularity and security. He then finds himself almost in a marginal man status where he is no longer a child but not yet an adult. The adolescent faces the increasing rapidity of physiological changes and his burgeoning sexuality pressuring him internally, while the external world is demanding proficiency in peer relationships, independent behavior, and goal orientation toward a vocation. One of the great dichotomies of adolescence is that the adolescent is immersed in the question "Who am I?" while the adults in his world are immersed in the question "What are you going to be?"

The overwhelming sense of self-consciousness characteristic of most adolescents, coupled with the almost certain insecurities about the image of the new body he finds himself inhabiting, make this a time of great turmoil for most young people. When one considers how the so-called normal, healthy adolescent is usually significantly stressed by the onslaught of physiological, sexual, and psychological changes during adolescence, the effects of this difficult period on the terminally ill adolescent are indeed profound and far-reaching in their implications. The terminally ill adolescent's quest for independence is seriously abated by his unavoidable dependency on parents and other adults for his physical care, especially during periods of hospitalization. At a time when peer approval and body image are of heightened significance the adolescent with a terminal illness must deal with serious alterations in his physical appearance from medication, such as extreme hair loss, weight loss, or bloating. During adolescence a sense of alienation is inevitable. The terminal adolescent often encounters increased alienation of family and friends who are unable to respond appropriately to his needs. At a time when the adult world is asking "What are you going to be?" the terminally ill adolescent must contend with the reality that he probably won't survive long enough to answer that question for himself or others.

When an individual reaches adolescence his understanding of death is usually similar to that of the adult. During adolescence the magical thinking about death characteristic of childhood has declined and the adolescent's level of cognitive functioning enables him to perceive death in the adult conceptual framework of finality, permanence, and irreversibility.

Before turning to some of the literature on the terminally ill adolescent, an examination of the work of Dr. Elisabeth Kübler-Ross and Dr. Avery Weisman on terminal illness in adults offers some significant insights valuable in understanding the adolescent as well as adults.

Dr. Kübler-Ross's book *On Death and Dying* (1969) elucidates some of the concerns, needs, and dilemmas that the terminal patient encounters. In order to help us empathize with the intensity of grief that a dying person faces, she asks people to imagine the trauma and tragedy of losing one beloved person. She then goes on to stress the enormity of the grieving response of the dying person who is about to lose everyone and everything that he has ever loved and cherished throughout his life. Dr. Ross believes that patients usually know when they have a serious illness and that they have a right to be told as long as the person telling them allows for some hope and makes a commitment not to desert the patient. This is not to say that false hope should be given, but rather a statement that perhaps something unforeseen such as a new cure may occur so that they may live longer than expected or have a remission. In her extensive work with terminal patients Dr. Ross has found that people usually welcome the opportunity to speak candidly about their feelings about dying.

Dr. Ross's book delineates five stages of emotional responses to terminal illness that usually occur in a patient. The stages are not always sequential, sometimes overlap, and a person can move back and forth from one stage to another. The first stage of response upon learning about terminal illness is that a person will react with shock and denial. Dr. Ross believes that when family, friends, or hospital staff can genuinely convey to the person that they are ready to talk about the illness, this helps the patient to drop his denial and move into the next stage which is anger. This is the time when the patient usually experiences a necessary and appropriate rage, hostility, and overwhelming sense of helplessness. The next stage is bargaining, where the person often will make some promise in exchange for prolongation of life. The next stage is depression, when the patient acknowledges the reality of his circumstances. Dr. Ross contends that at this point the patient is engaging in preparatory grief and has a right to do so. The fifth stage of acceptance, which is not resignation by any means, occurs when the patient feels he has finished his unfinished business and is now ready to meet his imminent death. Dr. Ross contends that a patient who has been allowed to express his feelings honestly can enter acceptance with a genuine sense of peacefulness.

Dr. Weisman of the Harvard Medical School has also made noteworthy contributions in the treatment of terminal patients. In his book *On Dying and Denying* (1972) he defines three psychosocial stages of responses that the terminal patient passes through as the severity of his physiological condition increases. The first stage is Primary Recognition which covers the time from the patient's first recognition that something is wrong until the time of the definitive medical diagnosis. During this stage most patients display denial and postponement. Stage two is termed Established Disease and covers the period from a patient's initial response to his diagnosis and his reactions prior to the onset of the terminal period. This stage usually finds the patient dealing with his illness by varying degrees of mitigation and displacement of death concerns. The third stage of Final Decline begins when the patient has reached the terminal stage and begins the decline toward death and ends when death is at hand. During this period the patient must compromise his autonomy due to the gravity of his physical condition; yet it is imperative that he have a support system that allows him to maintain his dignity, decency, and self-respect.

The adolescent's cognizance of death parallels the adult's in many ways. Therefore, it may be beneficial to examine the terminal adolescent's affective responses in terms of Dr. Ross's paradigm. Also, Dr. Weisman's model of the emotional concomitants of progressive states of physical decline can provide further insights into the issues the adolescent with a terminal illness faces. However, it is important to note that due to the fact that an adolescent is at a critical stage in his development, his response to a terminal illness will in certain ways differ from his adult counterpart.

In his work with terminal patients, Gullo (1973) has found certain coping patterns specifically characteristic of adolescents. Gullo defines seven coping patterns found in terminal adolescents and stresses the importance of helping professionals not imposing their philosophical persuasions upon patients by adhering to one coping style as superior to another. He contends that just as each young person lives in his unique way, he should be allowed to die in his unique way, selecting the coping style that enables him to adjust to his impending death.

One of the coping patterns, according to Gullo, seen in terminal adolescents is that of death acceptor. This adolescent acknowledges the reality of his illness, doesn't give up hope for life, yet doesn't deceive himself, and proceeds to make the adjustments of his continued illness. Almost antithetical to the death acceptor is the death denier who is often supported by his parents in denial of the existence or gravity of his illness. Gullo claims that as the illness progresses, maintenance of this coping mechanism becomes increasingly difficult. There is another type of death denier who admits to the gravity of his illness, yet insists that he will be the one to beat the odds and survive. Some adolescents respond to terminal illness as death submitters by viewing themselves as doomed, passive victims. Their overwhelming sense of helplessness results in gloom and pessimism. Another coping style is that of the death facilitator who consciously or unconsciously behaves in a way to abet his death. The range of behaviors may include such actions as refusal to take medicine or submit to medical treatments or direct suicide attempts. Another coping style is seen in the death transcender who goes beyond acceptance of death to view death in a broader context of existential or religious significance. Adherents to the death transcender coping style (who are few in number) still mourn and grieve, yet they seem to have internalized a value system that allows them to perceive the process of dying as a point on a spiritual or philosophic continuum. The death defier chooses another response to his circumstances by refusing to "give in" to death although he recognizes the severity of his illness. Although these adolescents really don't expect their arduous struggles to save them, their efforts are geared toward maintaining their self-respect and dignity and expressing their rage.

Usually, whether a terminal adolescent's coping mechanisms are successful in reducing anxiety is inextricably woven into the coping behaviors of his family. In her work with terminal adolescents and their families, Lowenberg (1970) classifies coping behaviors into two categories. On the one hand are the approach behaviors which work toward restitution and acceptance of the reality of the illness. On the other hand are the avoidance or denial behaviors. Lowenberg contends that at certain stages in terminal illness denial is appropriate, adaptive behavior. However, she believes that denial behaviors must be given up, at least partially, at a certain point to allow the adolescent and his family the opportunity to do the anticipatory work of grieving that facilitates healthier adjustment for all concerned. Included in avoidance behaviors are hostility toward staff, intellectualizing about details of the disease, avoidance of discussion of death, parental avoidance of the patient, overactivity, failure to exhibit affect during discussions of the illness, social isolation, self-punitive attitudes, fantasizing, excessive dependence on religion, and unrealistic plans for the distant future. Among the approach behaviors are present orientation, planning for time of death and afterward, discussing death openly, freely expressing sorrow and depression, crying, parental acknowledgment that the adolescent is aware of the situation, reviewing the past, behavior indicating appropriate cognitive perception of the illness, seeking help, turning to religion, and verbalizing about previous affective states of nonacceptance.

In their work with leukemic children and their families at Los Angeles County—U.S.C. Medical Center (1971) Kaplan, Smith, Grobstein, and Fischman found that a family's ability to manage their child's terminal illness is dependent on both parents resolving the coping tasks of diagnosis early in the crisis. Among the maladaptive family coping styles which impede this imperative early resolution is gross denial of the diagnosis. Such families will refrain from referring to the illness as "leukemia," using such terms as virus, anemia, or blood disease. Such parents often cling to the possibility of a wrong diagnosis, yet rarely do they deny their children medical treatment. These parents often go to extreme precautions to prevent revelation of the diagnosis, usually erroneously fearing that the truth would cause mental breakdown or suicide. Another form of denial behavior in parents is "flights into activity" such as a new pregnancy or moving. Those parents who deny the diagnosis often will display hostility toward the hospital staff.

Some parents will accept the diagnosis of leukemia but refuse to accept the prognosis of the disease as incurable or fatal, even when the course of their child's illness confirms the disease as terminal. Such parents often shop for exotic cures, try to treat the disease through diets, or resort to faith healing. Still another group of parents may accept the diagnosis and the prognosis of the illness, yet abdicate care of the child. These parents may abandon their children during hospitalization, claiming there is nothing they can do to help the child. Still another maladaptive parental coping behavior is what these researchers term discrepant parental coping, which occurs when the parents exhibit opposing positions in their coping mechanisms.

Literature on terminal illness in all age groups confirms that the patient's coping mechanisms can be either helped or hindered by the coping skills of his family. The ambivalent position of the adolescent as neither child nor adult in the family unit, along with the normal tension associated with facing adolescent developmental tasks, can make this an extremely stressful period of family relationships. When the trauma of terminal illness is added to this already difficult period, the result can be that the family undergoes an extremely disintegrative experience. The literature suggests the crucial significance of early intervention in helping the family develop coping behaviors that will facilitate both the patient's and the family's facing the reality of what lies ahead. Although there is some disagreement among researchers in terms of how long denial behaviors should be maintained, there is agreement that both the patient and his family can be moved forward toward acceptance when helping professionals can speak with them openly and honestly about death. The literature continually reaffirms that as a prerequisite for working with terminal patients the helper must first have resolved his own fears and anxieties about death.

For two semesters I spent one day a week working with children and adolescents, many of whom were terminally ill, at Childrens Hospital therapeutic playrooms. From my practical experience and research, I believe that the developmental tasks of adolescence can be utilized to facilitate successful coping with terminal illness. One of the most essential tasks the adolescent faces is assertion of his autonomy and independence. Resolution of this task is not easy when the adolescent has a terminal illness and must be hospitalized or confined to bed rest for long periods of time. I believe that a way to allow the adolescent to assert his independence within the parameters of his dependency on others for physical care is through involvement in helping relationships where he is the helper. During periods of hospitalization this could involve assigning a younger child with a terminal illness to the adolescent. The adolescent, at the appropriate time, could take a major part in explaining medical procedures to the child and sharing his feelings and experience of the illness. The adolescent could also be present during treatments as a support system for the child. The relationship could be continued outside the hospital by giving the adolescent clearly defined responsibilities such as weekly phone calls to the child. The adolescent could also be assigned tasks in writing about his illness and medical procedures for a hospital handbook for younger children.

I feel that group sessions for adolescents are essential in helping them make peer adjustments. In a group setting they can on the one hand form a peer group who shares their concerns and on the other hand have an opportunity to deal with the many trying and painful circumstances they are facing with their healthy peers at school. In such a setting the terminal adolescent can discover that he is not alone in his problems at home and school. A technique that I believe would be especially efficacious in such a group setting would be extensive use of role playing of situations the terminally ill adolescent must face, such as embarrassing questions about altered physical appearances.

One of the issues that distinguishes adolescence from childhood is that the adolescent is beginning to deal with futuristic thinking and goal setting. I believe that the terminally ill adolescent should participate in this task. However, he should be assisted by his family and helping professionals in setting continuing short-term, yet challenging, goals rather than distant, unrealistic goals. No terminal patient should be deprived of hope. In my view, when the adolescent's support systems do not attend to the crucial task of assisting him in setting realistic, attainable goals, they are giving a clear message of resignation that will probably result in his loss of hope. I observed at Childrens Hospital how important it was to the children and adolescents to continue with schoolwork, even during the final stages of the terminal phase of their illness. For these individuals school was associated with the future and hope, and continued participation was a successful means of coping.

One of the most obvious manifestations of the adolescent's cognitive functioning is the characteristic questioning of values, philosophizing and intellectualizing. During adolescence existential and spiritual issues are often probed with an intense ardor. I believe that this tendency which many adolescents manifest could, under the proper guidance, greatly assist the adolescent in coping with his terminal illness. There are a multiplicity of ways that this could be accomplished. One way would be to have group sessions for adolescents with religious leaders or philosophy professors to openly discuss concepts of death, dying, and afterlife. Another way would be to have workshops in poetry, journal keeping, short story, and play writing given by professionals in these fields. An important aspect of dealing with this task is to give the adolescent a forum for expression of his views. This could take such forms as a poetry anthology to be distributed to fellow patients. A method of giving those adolescents who wish to share their views verbally would be to ask them to lecture to students in the helping professions about these issues.

In my view, the thesis of Viktor Frankl's book, *Man's Search for Meaning* (1959), has special significance for the terminal adolescent and his family. Frankl contends that even in the most tragic circumstances there is one freedom that can never be taken away from a person—the ability to choose the attitude with which he faces the circumstances he must endure. Even in the midst of extreme suffering, a person can find meaning in his life if he can find meaning in his suffering. Frankl quotes Nietzsche to make this point: "He who has a why to live can bear almost any how." I feel that therapeutic interventions with the terminal adolescent and his family should focus upon Frankl's principles of logotherapy which seek to aid people in rising above their outward fate by finding a purpose in their suffering.

I believe that if interventions can be made with a terminal child and his family to establish successful coping behaviors and to discover a meaning in their suffering, the adolescent's terminal illness can be an integrative rather than disintegrative experience for all concerned. I would like to share a personal experience to make this point. Last year at Childrens Hospital I became friends with a fifteen-year-old boy who was terminally ill. His name was Scott Ipswitch. On April 16, 1976, he died of Stage Four Hodgkin's disease and leukemia. Three nights before he died he asked to see me and I had the privilege of spending several hours alone with him. He chose to bear his pain silently and with a sense of humor. At one point he looked at me and said, "At this point I just want to make it as easy on everyone as possible." He asked me to make sure and read his private journals that he had kept over the years of his illness in doing research for my dissertation and told me that he was sure I'd get my doctorate. There was not much happiness in that hospital room that night but there was a sense of peace emanating from Scott which filled me with a mixture of serenity and sadness. Scott was blessed with a family who displayed many of the successful coping behaviors previously mentioned in this paper. His family helped him in the difficult task of finding meaning in his suffering. He left behind this poem as a reminder to all of us that even in the most painful of circumstances a personal meaning of life can be found.

> Proudly, majestically, I leave.
> Happy, content, I leave.
> I have done what I could to the end,
> Never surrendering
> I leave.
> I leave, forever.
>
> SCOTT IPSWITCH

BIBLIOGRAPHY

FRANKL, VIKTOR E. *Man's Search for Meaning*. New York: Pocket Books, 1975.

FULTON, ROBERT. *Death and Identity*. New York: John Wiley and Sons, 1966.

GULLO, STEPHEN V. "Games Dying Children Play." *Medical Dimensions*, October 1973.

JACKSON, PAT LUDDER. "The Child's Developing Concept of Death: Implications for Nursing Care of the Terminally Ill." *Nursing Forum* 14, no. 2 (1975): 204–15.

KAPLAN, SMITH, GROBSTEIN, and FISCHMAN. "Coping with Childhood Leukemia: A Severe Family Crisis." Part I. Los Angeles County—U.S.C. Medical Center paper, April 1971.

KÜBLER-ROSS, ELISABETH. *On Death and Dying*. New York: The Macmillan Company, 1969.

LOWENBERG, JUNE S. "The Coping Behaviors of Fatally Ill Adolescents and Their Parents." *Nursing Forum* 9, no. 3 (1970): 269–87.

WEISMAN, AVERY D. *On Dying and Denying*. New York: Behavioral Publications, 1972.

Shortly after Scott's death, we received a letter from the executive director of Childrens Hospital, Henry B. Dunlap, which was another testimony to the fact that Scott did indeed accomplish something. His letter said in part:

> One of the reasons Scott was special to us was that he had the rare talent to communicate his feelings to those around him. Even more, he had the inner security to use that talent in an open and objective way.

He held a mirror up for all of us who serve children like him. It is a view of ourselves to be examined carefully for it gave us a rare glimpse of how we really are to those to whom it matters. He showed us our flaws and our beauty with a clarity and honesty that could not be denied. We did not like all we saw in his mirror, but we are the better for having seen it through him.